ARKANA

YOUR HANDS CAN HEAL

Ric Weinman incorporates many forms of healing in his work as a spiritual therapist. In addition to the channelling methods taught in this book, he uses Jin Shin Jyutsu, cranial-sacral therapy, FasciaUnwinding™, visceral release, and emotional-body work. He teaches Energy Channelling/Aura Balancing Workshops, FasciaUnwinding™ Workshops, and Inner-Transformational Workshops based on the material in his second book, *One Heart Laughing*. He currently lives and practices healing in Tucson.

Ric A. Weinman

YOUR
HANDS
CAN
HEAL

Learn to Channel Healing Energy

EXPANDED EDITION

ARKANA

ARKANA
Published by the Penguin Group
Viking Penguin, a division of Penguin Books USA Inc.,
375 Hudson Street, New York, New York 10014, U.S.A.
Penguin Books Ltd, 27 Wrights Lane,
London W8 5TZ, England
Penguin Books Australia Ltd, Ringwood,
Victoria, Australia
Penguin Books Canada Ltd, 10 Alcorn Avenue, Suite 300,
Toronto, Ontario, Canada M4V 3B2
Penguin Books (N.Z.) Ltd, 182–190 Wairau Road,
Auckland 10, New Zealand

Penguin Books Ltd, Registered Offices:
Harmondsworth, Middlesex, England

First published in the United States of America by E. P. Dutton, a division of
NAL Penguin Inc., 1988
This revised edition published in Arkana Books 1992

1 3 5 7 9 10 8 6 4 2

A NOTE TO THE READER: The ideas, procedures, and suggestions contained in this book are not
intended as a substitute for consulting with your physician. All matters regarding your health
require medical supervision.

LIBRARY OF CONGRESS CATALOGING IN PUBLICATION DATA
Weinman, Ric A.
Your hands can heal
Bibliography: p.
1. Imposition of hands—Therapeutic use.   2. Force
and energy   3. Chakras.   I. Title.
RZ999. W44 1988
615.5   87–22358
ISBN 0 14 019.361 8(pbk.)

Printed in the United States of America
Illustrations by Shelley Kaniss

for Mary,

who taught me about silence
and unconditional love

CONTENTS

I

THREE METHODS FOR CHANNELLING
HEALING ENERGY

II

CREATING AN IN-DEPTH AURA BALANCING

III

THE FOURTH WAY

PREFACE

Channelling healing energy, also called "laying on of hands," is a form of healing that has always been shrouded in mystery. On the one hand, Western science, encountering a phenomenon that it couldn't explain, either declared that the phenomenon simply didn't exist or, when confronted with clear evidence that healing did indeed occur, simply declared that any "psychosomatic" illness could be cured by an "act of faith." And since, on the other hand, most healers themselves could not explain what they did and attributed the phenomenon to their faith in a deity, channelling healing energy was relegated to the realm of religion and labeled "faith healing." But this is a misnomer. For even atheists can be healed and learn to become healers. The channelling of healing energy is a phenomenon that is as natural and real as magnetism; it exists independently of the beliefs of participants or observers.

In the 1930s, a Russian scientist by the name of Semyon Davidich Kirlian began the first serious experiments with a photographic process that could capture images of the "aura"—the energy field around the body. When healers have their hands photographed with what is now called "Kirlian photography," there is a marked change in the image when they begin to channel healing energy. Where the photographs had shown smooth contours around the fingers, they now show long streams of light emanating from the hands and fingers. Clearly, something very concrete happens when people channel healing energy.*

One of the most amazing things about channelling healing energy is that as mysterious as it seems, and in spite of the small number of healers who practice this form of healing, it can be taught to almost anyone. The process of channelling healing energy is so natural and innate that once the principles and methods are explained it is very easy to learn. Even if you've never experienced anything esoteric, and whether you believe in God or not, you can learn to channel healing energy.

This book is based on energy channelling/aura balancing workshops that I have taught in Tucson, Arizona, and New York City. In these workshops, people of all ages have learned—by the end of the first day—to channel healing energy in three completely different ways. So, if you think you won't be able to learn how to channel healing energy, put your worries aside. At least one of these methods will work for you, and you will be surprised at how easy it is.

There are many advantages in learning how to channel

---

*Kirlian photography uncovered the equally concrete "phantom leaf effect." Sometimes, when part of a leaf is cut away and the remaining part is photographed using Kirlian methods, the aura of the entire leaf appears in the photograph. (This may explain why people sometimes feel pain in missing limbs.) A similar phenomenon is found in Kirlian photographs of germinating seeds: the root tips sometimes appear in the photographs before they manifest physically. These phenomena have finally convinced many scientists that there is an aura associated with living things.

healing energy in a workshop. One is the experience of learning and sharing with others. Another is that healers who run such workshops are "in tune" enough with energy to see what you are doing and to demonstrate how you might work more effectively or more powerfully. If you have trouble at any point, the healer can quickly help you through it. Also, when many people are channelling energy together, the energy is easier to channel.

But there are very few places in the world today where a person can go to learn how to channel healing energy. And even these are hard to find. Many of my workshops, for instance, draw people solely by word of mouth. Because of this scarcity of learning centers and because I believe it is time for people to have access to this information, I have written this book. In this age of spiralling medical costs, people are ready to learn how to heal themselves and one another. Also, as people practice channelling healing energy, they expand their awareness and transform their lives. I believe that many people are ready for this kind of personal and spiritual growth. Everywhere I go, I meet people who have only recently awakened to the immense possibilities for personal growth that are available to them.

INTRODUCTION

The channelling of healing energy occurs when one allows oneself to be a vehicle, or channel, through which healing energy can flow. This healing energy can cure physical diseases by releasing the stress and long-held emotional traumas that are the root causes of disease. Healing energy can have such a profound effect because everything in the universe is made up of energy. Einstein proved this mathematically with his famous equation $E = mc^2$, which states that all matter, from the atom to the elephant, is made up of energy. Even stress, disease, and emotional traumas are forms or patterns of energy. Therefore they can all be affected by energy (including channelled healing energy) and changed by it. (See Appendix B: "An Alternative Theory of Disease.")

My goal in this book is to give you a very broad experience of working with healing energy—an experience broad enough for you to take what you learn here and be creative with it on your own. You will learn three very different methods for channelling healing energy through your hands as well as two methods for channelling healing energy from a distance; you will learn how to use healing energy to clear chakras and create an in-depth aura balancing; and you will learn a non-channelling way of healing that I call "healing through Oneness." By the time you finish this book you will be able to be a channel for any healing vibration you are familiar with.

Yet all the healing methods you will learn here are *tools*. Healing itself—how you use those tools—is ultimately an art. Healing always involves sharing, and no one will ever be able to completely systematize the love or creativity of the heart.

THREE

NOTES ON

USING THIS

BOOK

1. It is important to use this book in sequence, because each exercise requires the knowledge gained from those preceding it.

2. Although this book is based on my two-day weekend workshops, I strongly suggest that you do not try to learn it all from the book in a single weekend. Here are two suggested learning schedules:

FOUR EVENINGS AND ONE DAY

    First evening: Chapters 1 and 2 (including the Warm-Up Exercise and Exercises 1 and 2)

    Second evening: Chapter 3

    Third evening: Chapter 4

    Fourth evening: Chapters 5, 6, 7, and 8 (including Exercises 3 and 4)

    Saturday or Sunday: Chapters 9, 10, and 11 (including Exercises 5 and 6 and aura balancing), and Chapter 12 (optional)

A DAY, AN EVENING, AND A SECOND DAY

First day: Chapters 1, 2, 3, and 4 (including the Warm-
Up Exercise and Exercises 1 and 2)

Evening (on a different day): Chapters 5, 6, 7, and 8 (including Exercises 3 and 4)

Second day: Chapters 9, 10, and 11 (including Exercises
5 and 6 and aura balancing), and Chapter 12 (optional)

The first schedule would be ideal for most people. The evenings could be spread out over the week, building up learning
and awareness until the complete aura balancing is performed
on the weekend. Except for people with unusual schedules or
with a three-day weekend, the second schedule would leave
gaps of several days in the continuum of the learning, since
there would be only one evening session between the first
weekend day and the following weekend day. This could be
offset, though, if one or two evenings were used to practice
what had been learned, maintaining the level of awareness.

3. Because channelling healing energy usually involves a
second person, who is the recipient of the energy, a partner
is needed for you to practice and learn with. Therefore, all
the exercises in this book are designed for two people.* (Or
you can form a learning group with several twosomes.) If only
one of the two people is learning how to channel, the other
can simply receive. Learning is enhanced, though, if both
people are learning how to channel. Then each can experience
both sides of the healing situation, the channelling as well as
the receiving. The opportunity should not be missed to learn

---

*Although some of the channelling exercises are set up for both people to
learn the channelling at the same time, you may find it easier to take turns
so that one can read the directions while the other learns to channel.

firsthand what the receiver experiences. Also, if you learn to channel healing energy with someone else, you will have someone to compare your own experiences with.

WARM-UP EXERCISE:

CENTERING

THROUGH RECEIVING

THE BREATH

When acting as a channel for healing energy, it helps to be centered within oneself, experiencing the abundance of Life. To accomplish this, we simply *receive our breath*. Our breath is always here and now, and when we consciously receive our breath, we experience the abundance of Life, for breath *is* the gift of Life. In fact, it is an unconditional gift, for it does not depend on our thoughts or behavior; we only need to receive it. (When we tighten ourselves and restrict our breath, we block our capacity to receive Life, creating an inner sense of lack or loss or neediness.)

So, close your eyes, and for ten minutes consciously receive your breath. Receive it into the core of your being and into every cell of your body. You never have to "take" a breath; simply receive the breath that has already been given to you and allow it to fill you with Life. (If you encounter an area within yourself where you have difficulty receiving, don't try to force the breath there, simply be willing to receive your breath in that place.)

Utilize this exercise briefly before beginning each of the other exercises in this book and before any healing session. It can also be used as a regular meditation.

YOUR
HANDS
CAN
HEAL

I

THREE
METHODS FOR
CHANNELLING
HEALING
ENERGY

1

DOORWAYS
TO ENERGY
SOURCES

The world in which we live is composed entirely of energy. We are forever immersed in and surrounded by energy. The first important question is, how do we get access to some of that energy so we can make use of it? It turns out that there are many ways, and we can use all of them: our minds, our imaginations, our memories, our fantasies, our emotions, and our bodies. They are all doorways to sources of healing energy.

Part of the secret of channelling healing energy is allowing yourself to feel connected to a source of positive energy and then allowing that energy to flow through you so you can share it with someone else. With all the methods of energy channelling that I teach, you are not *doing* the channelling, you are *allowing it to happen*. The energy is actually channelling itself. You are simply the vehicle or channel through which it moves. And the source of that energy can be anything that makes you feel wonderful, for when you feel wonderful you are allowing yourself to receive energy from some kind of positive, healing source.

Most of us, at some point in our lives, have had an experience in which we were flooded with so much happiness that we were almost overcome by it. That memory is a doorway to a positive energy source. Most of us have had fantasies that momentarily inspired us with an incredible sense of joy. These fantasies are doorways to sources of positive energy. We will use these memories and fantasies when we come to the third method of channelling.

Another way to connect to a healing energy source is to tap various energy centers within or outside of the body. These centers are natural doorways to sources of positive energy. When we feel love for someone, the energy center in the area of the heart pours out energy. When we feel sexually attracted to someone, the energy center in the area of the pelvis pours out a different kind of energy. (That's one way we know when someone is strongly attracted to us: we can feel the energy from their sexual center touching us, and we recognize the kind of energy it is.) There are other energy centers, and we will use some of them in the first two methods of channelling.

Words are also doorways to energy sources. Because we associate words with the experiences they represent, the use of those words tends to make us remember those experiences and re-create them in the present. In a sense, words are packages that contain pictures and feelings. Just saying some words will make us feel good, while others can make us feel ill. If we say the word "hate" over and over in our minds for an hour, we will probably become physically ill. The repetition of the word "love," on the other hand, will make us feel relaxed and peaceful. The word "love" automatically connects us to the energy source that love is. Words, therefore, can be used to make a connection to particular energy sources or to maintain a connection to one.

Colors, too, are sources of positive energy, and each color is the source of a different kind of energy. Staring at the color red or visualizing it internally will create a very different feeling and energy state than doing the same thing with the color green. Later we will discuss the effects and meaning of the different colors, for each color has a different effect upon the body.

Traditionally, religious feelings have been the most common energy source for channelling healing energy. Those who feel a deep connection to God, Jesus, Buddha, or a spiritual teacher can use that feeling as an energy source in the third method of channelling.

Perhaps the ultimate way of connecting to a positive, healing energy source lies in perceiving the present moment in such a way as to automatically fill you with happiness and joy. Then life itself is your energy source and you are filled with its energy constantly. Learning this way, of course, is the most difficult. Usually only people who are deeply involved in a religious or spiritual discipline will come to this experience. Yet it is a possibility that is open to all of us. For, independent of religious or spiritual beliefs, what creates this state of mind more readily than anything else is the simple, nonsectarian practice of unconditional love. And as we will see in the next chapter, unconditional love has a central, even if sometimes hidden, role to play in all methods of channelling healing energy.

EXERCISE 1: COLORS, WORDS, AND MEMORIES

Both people should sit on chairs facing each other, several feet apart. (If there is a group, make a circle.) These should not be soft armchairs, but rather chairs that are fairly easy to sit up straight in. Pick one person to lead the exercise, which has two parts.

First, close your eyes and take a minute to center yourself through receiving your breath. Then, eyes still closed, whoever is leading says the name of a color. Both people then say it silently (in your minds) while visualizing and feeling the color. Also, try breathing the color into your body. Just imagine that instead of breathing air, you are breathing light—whatever color light you are working with. Then, after half a minute of being absorbed with this color, the leader will name another one. Go through as many colors as you like, being sure to include blue, green, yellow, red, orange, gold, white, pink, black, and violet, not necessarily in that order. Notice your experience with each color.

When you have finished with the colors, do the same thing with various emotions, making sure to include "positive" as well as "negative" emotions. Sometimes it helps to say the word loudly in your mind, rather than softly. Allow yourself to feel whatever experience these words create for you.

Finally, do the same thing with concept words, such as home, music, mother, father, resistance, surrender, light, dark, God, earth, sky, beauty, creativity, freedom, choking, death, sweet, terror, and so on. Ten words will be sufficient. Allow yourself to experience whatever feelings these words create for you.

When you have finished, discuss your experiences with your partner. And remember, there is no "right" experience. Whatever you experienced is just what you experienced. It's important to be honest and not make judgments (different from perceptions) about your experience.

For the second part, allow about four feet of space between your chairs. Now, each of you should remember the highest, happiest, brightest, most ecstatic moment of your life. It can be the moment you felt the most love or the most alive. Use as many of your senses as you can to remember it, and try to re-create that feeling right now. Before you stop, pick a key word or image that will help you to get back to and re-create this state more quickly the next time.

If you can't remember a moment of such happiness, create a fantasy situation. Make it as intense as you can. Allow yourself to surrender to the fantasy and really experience it. Find a word that will enable you to re-create the feeling of this fantasy later on.

When you are done, share your experiences with your partner.

One purpose of this exercise is to show you how words, colors, feelings, memories, and your five senses can all be used to create particular internal energy states. The other purpose is to put you in tune with subtle shifts of energy and to give you a sense of the infinitely various forms that energy states may take. Channelling those energy states to energize or heal someone is just a few short steps away.

2

MIND-SET

The most important thing to learn if you are going to act as a healer is the healing mind-set. Your attitude, your frame of mind, the way you view and approach the healing situation, is critical. Throughout this book I will remind you of this, and yet as much as I will stress it, I cannot stress it enough: *Your mind-set is the most important thing to remember in any healing situation.*

There are six attitudes to be aware of for creating the healing mind-set:

1. *Sharing Healing Energy with vs. Doing Healing On.* Although the appearance of any energy channelling situation is that a healer is doing something *to* or *on* someone, this is not the case. The healer is doing something *with* the other person. This may seem to be a subtle difference, but it is actually a very important one because it affects the healer's attitude towards the other person and towards the healing sit-

uation in general. If I am doing healing *on* someone, then there is a certain kind of separateness in my attitude. The other person will be seen as a neutral and passive aspect of a situation in which I have all the responsibility and am doing all the work. On the other hand, if I am sharing energy *with* someone, then we are both responsible for what is happening, and the success or failure of what we attempt will depend upon our mutual openness to the experience. With sharing, I will tend to view what is happening in terms of "us" rather than "me/ you." This will make me feel much more connected to the person I am working with and much more open to him or her. It will also create more awareness of what is happening to that person and where the real problems lie. Finally, sharing helps me to experience the other person as my equal and prevents my ego from getting in the way.

2. *Equality vs. Ego Power Trips.* In every healing situation there will be an interaction between two people. One person will play the role of healer and the other the role of receiver. At the end, both will have benefited from the interaction, whether that be healing, or learning, or some other kind of experience. In a sense, you are both students of the situation. Your roles are different, but you are *equal*. You are both human beings who have come together, each for your own personal reasons, to share a healing situation. This is very important because it is easy for the person who is playing the role of healer to get caught up in his ego and develop what are called "power trips" with respect to the other person. Some doctors are known to treat their patients in this way. They deal with their patients as objects or nonpeople without realizing that, as a result, they also turn themselves into nonpeople and erect barriers to the healing process. In every healing situation two individuals come together to create personal experiences for themselves. There is a basic equality, even though each

plays a different role. If one ego, to inflate itself, sees the other as less than equal, certain problems will be created, especially the problem of "trying to."

3. *No Trying To's.* Channelling healing energy means that you become a *vehicle* for healing energy to flow through you. It is not you in the sense of your ego that does the healing; it is the energy that is moving through you. And you don't have to do anything to have this energy move through you. All you need is an awareness of the energy and a willingness to allow it to work. Your role has quite a bit of passivity to it. The more you can just *be* with the energy, as opposed to trying to make it work, the fewer unconscious barriers you will put up and the more powerful the energy can be. While the ego is a natural part of us, the problem it creates for healing is that it wants to "do" and be in control. It doesn't realize that its "doings" get in the way of the flow of the energy. All of the ego's "trying to's"—really a form of resisting life as it is— create a tight whirlwind of activity that blocks the energy; the energy needs relaxedness, openness, and space in order to flow. In addition, if the ego thinks it is responsible for what is happening, it will become very attached to the results. This, too, will block energy flow, for if what the ego expects isn't happening, it will automatically try harder, and trying will always block energy flow. Since the energy that heals does not come from the ego, the ego cannot make it flow. It is not responsible for the healing. It is also not responsible when healing does not occur.* In the role of healer, you need to *allow* energy to flow, not try to cause it to happen.

---

*Healing is a mutual process. *No one can be healed of something they are not willing to let go of*. The healer is responsible for channelling the clearest energy possible. Ultimately, though, it is the other person who decides (usually unconsciously) how that healing energy will be used and whether or not healing will actually take place.

4. *No Judgments.* Any judgments you make about another person tend to create separation and foster a "me/you" attitude. Most judgments (as opposed to perceptions, which have no moralizing content) are nothing more than reflections of our own self-righteousness. Needless to say, this does not help energy flow. Judgments come from the ego, which enjoys feeling better and "more right" than other people. Since we all make judgments out of habit, if you hear your mind make a judgment, you can just take note of it without identifying or agreeing with it. Then the judgment has no power over you or any power to block your energy; it is just a passing thought.

5. *Connectedness.* There are two ways to perceive connectedness. Use the one that works best for you (or use both). The first is to use the perspective that, since we are all human beings, we are a family. All other human beings are literally your sisters and brothers. If you perceive someone as part of your family, related to you, you will feel a sense of connectedness you would not feel otherwise. The second way to perceive connectedness is to understand that we are all different forms of energy. While it is easy to tell one form from another (a rock is not a tree), the energy that makes up each form is the same. Whether you call this energy "God," the "Is" of existence, or just Energy, we are all created from this same energy, and this energy is ultimately who we are. This means that on our deepest level, on the level where our being is this energy, we are also all the forms that are created out of it, and all the forms are absolutely connected. In practical terms, this means that when we work with someone, we're really just helping another part of ourselves.*

The perception of connectedness is very important, for it

---

*This idea is the basis of the fourth way of healing: "healing through Oneness."

maintains our awareness of equality, helps to keep the ego out of the picture, and creates a deep sense of openness to the other person. And if you encounter a person with your heart open, without ego, with no judgments, and with a sense of "us," the feeling that will almost certainly arise is unconditional love.

6. *Unconditional Love.* Unconditional love arises automatically from the practice of the first five attitudes. It is also a shortcut: the practice of unconditional love creates and maintains the other five attitudes. When we feel unconditional love for a person, there are no judgments, no trying to's, no sense of inequality, no perception of the other person as a nonperson, and there is a feeling of connectedness. Unconditional love is not something that has to be created. *Unconditional love already exists.* It is simply hidden under the layers of our fears, needs, desires, judgments, trying to's, and so on. So you don't need to create unconditional love; you only need to find the place inside yourself where it already exists. Unconditional love sees the person rather than that person's behavior. If you are spiritually oriented, unconditional love sees the pure, loving, spiritual being inside the forgetfulness of the human condition. When you feel unconditional love for someone, you have bypassed all the outer layers of their (and your) personality, including the "negative" aspects, the masks, and the fears. You have created a direct connection with who they really are, a connection that is free of ego and pretension. Unconditional love, therefore, is the perfect key for any healing situation. It automatically establishes the healing mind-set for channelling healing energy. It is *in itself* healing, and is ultimately the basis for all healing. Unconditional love goes right to the source. If you practice it, not only will your healing work be very powerful, but you will transform your own life as well.

EXERCISE 2: UNCONDITIONAL LOVE

This is a 'three-part exercise. Sit on chairs facing each other and close enough so that you can hold each other's hands comfortably. One person will be referred to as A, and the other as B. Choose beforehand which one you will be.

1. (Five minutes.) *Person A:* Close your eyes, extend your awareness, and sense what you can about your partner's body, mind, or feelings (even if you don't think you can do this).

Person B: Close your eyes and simply be neutral.

2. (Five minutes.) *Person A:* Without touching your partner, create within yourself the first five attitudes of the healing mind-set, just as if you were about to begin a healing session with this person. In this mind-set, you experience yourself about to share healing energy *with* your partner rather than doing healing *on her,** and you feel a sense of equality with your partner—you're two individuals playing different roles in a healing session. You are also not trying to prove anything; there is no ego involved. Clear your mind of any judgments. Just accept your partner as she is and see if you can experience a sense of connectedness on some level.

Person B: While your partner is establishing his mind-set, you are just sitting and receiving. This means that you are not trying to do anything, but are just open to experience whatever (if anything) happens.

3. (Ten minutes.) *Person A:* Having created the first five attitudes of the proper mind-set, now focus on the place within yourself where you feel unconditional love for your partner. If this feeling already came up in the last part of the exercise,

---

*In the various exercises throughout this book, I have tried to alternate use of the personal pronouns. In some instances the receiver, or partner, is female, in others male, and likewise for the channeller.

just continue to focus on it. As you get in touch with this place and this feeling, direct this feeling towards your partner and touch her with it. In other words, feel yourself actually sharing this love with her. This doesn't involve any trying to's, though. Just allow yourself to be open enough to share the unconditional love you are feeling. To send more love, simply allow yourself to experience more love and share more love. Remember that you don't have to create unconditional love; all you have to do is allow yourself to touch the place where it already exists within you.

Person B: You just sit and receive, without expectations, open to whatever you might experience.

4. (Ten minutes.) For this last part, both of you do exactly what you were doing before, but this time Person A holds his partner's hands. In addition, while you are mentally sharing unconditional love with your partner, visually imagine and feel that this unconditional love is travelling down your arms and is going directly out from your hands into Person B. You don't have to *make* this happen, though. If you just imagine and feel it happening, and allow yourself to share in this way, it will happen automatically. Your intention will guide the energy flow.

Person B: You sit and receive whatever you experience, without expectations.

When you have finished, take a few minutes to stretch. Don't discuss what happened yet. When you've finished stretching, repeat the exercise with the roles reversed. Then discuss your experiences. Note the differences between your experiences of each part of the exercise. *Accept whatever your experience is.* If one person felt something when he was receiving and the other didn't, that's okay. If one person wasn't able to feel unconditional love for the other, that's okay too. It will get easier. At the same time, if there is an emotional block there, the block should be explored. (Any part of the exercise may be repeated if so desired.) Going over the attitudes of the mind-set, one by one, may help to uncover where the block is. Remember, unconditional love does not have to be created; it is already there. It does not come from the ego. It arises automatically from a deeper level when the first five attitudes of the healing mind-set are observed. Or more simply, it occurs when you are willing to touch the place within yourself where unconditional love exists.

Unconditional love is the true basis for all healing. It creates the proper mind-set for any channelling of healing energy, and in every channelling method it is the actual force beneath all the outer forms. Without unconditional love there would be no giving and sharing, which are essential for any healing to occur. And since unconditional love is the inner essence of all healing, it can be used directly as an energy source, as we will see in the third method of channelling.

It is important to remember that when you feel blocked from giving unconditional love, that block has nothing to do with the other person. Unconditional love is *un*conditional, independent of behavior. Therefore, *the block always and only has to do with yourself.* If you look carefully, you will find that whatever you can't accept or strongly dislike in another person is that which you have disowned or can't handle in yourself. The practice of unconditional love, therefore, is a continuous teaching; you are always being shown where *you* are stuck, which gives you the opportunity to transform and grow.

3

THE FIRST
METHOD OF
CHANNELLING
HEALING ENERGY

SOURCING FROM ABOVE

We all know that the earth has an atmosphere. We can't actually see it, but we have no doubt that it exists. And surrounding the earth, in addition to the air, is an electromagnetic field; that's why a compass points north. Bodies also have a kind of electromagnetic atmosphere around them. You can't usually see it, and it is harder to detect than the earth's atmosphere, but it's just as real. The word for that atmosphere is "aura," and as I described it in the Preface, it can be photographed by Kirlian photography.

Although I said that you usually can't see the aura, people who develop clairvoyant ability *can* see it. The halo that many people saw around Jesus' head was part of his aura. It was one of the energy centers in his aura. The more spiritually evolved a person is, the brighter this particular energy center becomes and the easier it is to see. The aura is made up of etheric energy and an electromagnetic field. More simply, it can be thought of as an "energy field" that both surrounds the body and pervades it. And just as the earth's atmosphere is much denser at low altitudes than at the top of a mountain, the aura, too, is much denser in the eighteen inches that are closest to the body than it is farther out. An awareness of the aura is important because when you channel healing energy for someone, you will be interacting quite a bit with her aura. In fact, channelling will probably make your hands sensitive enough to enable you to feel the person's aura as you channel for her.

In Chapter 11, when you learn to do an in-depth aura balancing, you will be working a lot with structures in the aura called "chakras." Chakras are simply energy centers which, like the aura, usually can't be seen. I'll discuss chakras later. For now it is enough to know that although the word "chakra" comes from the yogic disciplines of India, chakras themselves no more belong to the Eastern yogis than mathematics and science belong to the West. Independently of whatever country first discovered genes, you have them and they are yours. In the same way, all human beings have chakras independently of whoever discovered and named them.

The last important concept to grasp before learning how to channel healing energy is the law about the way this kind of energy works (like the laws about the way physical energy works). It says, very simply: *Energy follows thought*. This means that wherever you place your awareness and attention, consciously or unconsciously, energy will go there. An example of this is what happened in the last exercise: As you imagined (visually and with feelings) energy coming out of your hands, it did. Another example is the placebo effect: If people *think* they have been given an effective medicine their condition often improves, even when no medication was given. Energy follows thought. We will be using this concept a lot throughout the book.

THE PRINCIPLE OF THE FIRST METHOD

In this first method of channelling healing energy, we will make use of an energy center (a chakra) that exists eighteen inches to two feet above the head. Although this energy center is outside the body, it is still within your aura and is very much a part of you. It looks like a white sun. As you imagine and consciously visualize a white sun sitting eighteen inches to two feet directly above your head, the attention you bring to that area focuses awareness and energy into that energy center, waking it up and making it grow and glow more powerfully. In this method, you will be channelling the energy that comes out of this energy center. It is always functioning to some degree, but because energy follows thought, when you direct attention to it, you automatically feed it, opening it up and turning it more fully "on."

Each of the three methods of channelling energy draws on a particular type of energy. All of them are healing, and all of them are powerful. But each one has its own quality and strong point. If only one of these methods works easily for you, I'd suggest using that one all the time. But assuming some facility with all of them, often one kind of energy will be more appropriate than the others.

The first method of channelling uses an energy that has a quality of "white fire." It is therefore purifying and cleansing. If I want to detoxify someone or some part of him, or to "burn out" a cancer, this is the energy I would use. This energy is also the hardest and most forceful of the three energies. It therefore works best on soft conditions, like cancer, congestion, and grogginess. Muscular tension, on the other hand, is hard, so a soft energy would more easily penetrate it. The white fire, being harder, would tend to bounce off this kind of tension, but it sweeps away things that are soft. The key words for this energy are "force" and "purification."

DEVELOPING THE ENERGY

Both partners are going to learn how to do the basic channelling at the same time. Stand in a relaxed position with a generous amount of space between you, so your attention is not diverted by your awareness of the other person standing too close to you. (If you find it difficult to stand during any of these exercises, you may sit on a chair.) In the beginning you will have your eyes closed, and then at the very end, once the energy is fully moving, you will open them so you can practice channelling with your eyes open.

Step 1. Take your position, close your eyes, and take a minute to center yourself through receiving your breath. Do not worry about how your partner is doing; you will talk about your experiences when you are both done. Just be aware of yourself standing in the room with a nice-size square around you. When you feel relaxed, imagine that there is a white sun sitting eighteen inches to two feet directly above your head. Just stand with your arms at your sides, imagining this sun above your head. Feel its rays and its light pouring over you and going right through the top of your head, filling your head with light. Experience how wonderful its radiant light feels. If you are religious, you can imagine this light as God's light or God's love. You can also imagine it as that pure energy which fills all of creation. Or, as you visualize this white sun, you can just experience how wonderful its light feels without imagining it as anything other than what it is. Use whatever works best for you. If saying in your mind the words "white sun" helps you to maintain the visualization, you can do that, too.

Don't go on to Step 2 until you feel the energy of this sun around you and coming into your head. If you are having any trouble with this, imagine the sun a little higher above your head. (I suggest trying this in any case, to see if it makes the sensations of its light and energy any stronger.) Another thing to keep in mind is to stay relaxed. There are no trying to's here. Although you are actively imaging the sun, it is actually already there. Your visualization only helps you to become aware of it. And once you become aware of it, the amount of light that comes through depends more on how open you are to it—how much you can surrender to it—than on how hard you concentrate.*

Step 2. As your head fills with the sun's white light, feel the energy move down through your body, filling your torso, arms, and legs, and going right out your hands and the bottoms of your feet. It's important to feel the energy actually go out through your four extremities. And remember, as you are experiencing the light travelling through your body, keep your attention connected to the source of the light, the sun above your head. You are absorbing its radiance. Its light and energy are pouring over you and through you, purifying your body.

Step 3. When you can feel the sun's energy moving easily through your body and out your extremities, imagine the bottoms of your feet becoming closed, so that the energy goes down to your feet but not out the bottoms. All you have to do is visualize or feel this to have it happen; energy always follows thought.

Step 4. When you have closed the bottoms of your feet, hold your hands comfortably in front of you with the palms facing each other, approximately four to six inches apart. As you hold your hands like this, keeping your awareness connected to the sun above your head and imagining its energy going over and through your body, you should start to feel

---

*If you are one of those rare people who cannot easily channel energy sourced from above—your eighth chakra—just relax. The second method will probably work more easily for you.

a tingling in and between your hands. As you bring your awareness to this feeling (at the same time as you are keeping your awareness connected to the sun), the feeling will grow stronger. It may even get so strong that you will feel as if the energy would push your hands apart if you relaxed them. Stand for a few minutes in this energy flow. If you move your hands slightly back and forth, playing with the energy, you may develop a better feel for it. You might also try to see how far apart you can hold your hands and still feel the energy. Check occasionally to make sure the energy is also going down to your feet. The more of your body that is involved in the channelling, the more energy you will have available to you.

If at any point you lose the sense of the energy between your hands, relax and let go of any trying to's. Just allow the energy to be the way you are imagining it. Sometimes it helps to make sure you're not standing slumped over or pulled back; stand straight and allow yourself to relax. If the energy flow does not pick up, begin again at Step 1.

Step 5. When you feel the energy is well established, open your eyes and see if you can still maintain the awareness that keeps the energy flowing. See if you can maintain the energy flow while you are looking at things in the room.

Completion. When you can channel the energy easily with your eyes open, you may stop. And when you have both stopped, share (without competing) your experiences with each other. If you finish before your partner does, do not rush him. Give him as much time as he needs.

Awareness Note. With this method of channelling healing energy, remember to allow the sun's energy to come down to you rather than letting yourself float up to the sun. Your *awareness* goes up to the sun, but *you stay in your body.* This is a difficult point to explain if you have never experienced yourself "out of your body."* It has happened only twice in my workshops, so it is extremely rare and not something to worry about. If you should be one of the few people who float up to the sun and get out of their body, you will feel "spacy," a little seasick, or both. To release these symptoms, just sit down, extend your arms over your head, and imagine that you are grabbing hold of yourself and slowly pulling yourself down back into your head. Then sit with your hands on top of your head for a few minutes and the symptoms should disappear. If they do not, your partner can try gently pushing you back into your head. If the symptoms still persist, lie down for fifteen minutes with your partner holding (not squeezing) your big toes (to help reground you). If this, too, does not help, don't worry; you are in no danger and your symptoms will dissipate over the course of the day.

While you are channelling, if you feel the energy going all the way down to your feet, keeping you grounded, you won't have any "out of body" problems.

CHANNELLING THE SUN-ENERGY
TO ANOTHER PERSON

This form of channelling makes use of what I call a "field-charge." You build up an excess charge of positive healing energy in the energy field of your aura and share that extra charge with someone else. Since you develop this field-charge before you actually direct it towards anyone, at the time when you do direct it, your aura will be much more charged with positive energy than is the aura of the person who is receiving. Through this difference in charge, energy can be transferred or shared. But because concentrated and excess energy will

---

*Note: This is not the kind of "out of body" experience associated with astral travel.

tend to spread out into areas that have less energy, the transfer of charge can happen too quickly. Then the positive charge empties out of your charged auric field faster than your channelling can replace it. As a result, your charged field collapses, much as a balloon collapses when all the air goes out of it. Because the change occurs so suddenly, it may throw the electromagnetic field in your aura temporarily out of balance, making you feel tired and making it very difficult to re-create the channelling for a while. How long it will take for your aura to rebalance itself depends upon how radically you allowed your field to collapse. At the most it could take an hour or so, but field collapse will not be a problem if two simple precautions are taken.

PRECAUTIONS

1. When channelling from above, approach the other person's body *slowly*. Begin with your hands about a foot from your partner's head, and move slowly closer. This will enable you to control the rate at which healing energy is transferred to the other person. Transference actually begins whenever your two auras touch or whenever the energy coming out of your hands touches the other person's aura. But although auras normally extend for several feet from a body and can be much larger in a charged/channelling state, because the auras are relatively thin until you get close to the body, there isn't much contact or energy transference until you are physically close. At a foot's distance the aura is still pretty thin compared to the density in the last three inches. The most contact and transference occurs when you actually touch the other person's body. You will probably feel this shift in your partner's aura density as you slowly move closer with your channelling, but if you're not aware of it at first, don't worry; the sensitivity will come later.

2. Whenever you feel yourself losing your field-charge,

stop and clear yourself: step back a few feet, shake your hands, and reestablish the energy flow and field-charge. Then resume the channelling with your partner. The reason for shaking your hands is that when you pull your hands out of your partner's aura you will probably pull some "debris" out with you. This debris is the "negative" charges created by various forms of mental, emotional, and physical stress. The channelling clears out these negative charges, pushing some out the extremities and purifying others by charging them and turning them back into light. They stick to your hands for the same reason that water does when you put your hands in it, and for the same reason your hands smell of smoke if you put them over a fire. The debris in the aura, although invisible, has density and substance. When you pull your hands out of your partner's aura, some of it clings to you. It's nothing to be concerned about. Shaking your hands is simply an easy way to get rid of it. If you didn't shake your hands, when you resumed the channelling, you'd be putting the debris back into your partner's aura, and you'd then have that much more work to do to clear it out. So you want to shake your hands *away from* your partner.

After shaking your hands, since they will now be clear and unencumbered, a strong channelling should resume almost instantaneously. In addition, since you have pulled a hunk of negative charge out of your partner's aura, when you begin channelling into his head again, you will encounter less resistance than you did before. So it is helpful to periodically step back and shake your hands early on in the channelling when there's still a lot of negative charge in the other person's aura, even if you aren't losing your field-charge. Often the feeling of losing the field-charge is caused by nothing more than a lot of negative charge resisting the flow of your channelling. Getting rid of some of this resistance by pulling it out with your hands makes your channelling easier to move through your partner when you return to his aura, so your channelling will feel stronger. (This is especially true for the first method of channelling. Since it's a harder energy, it bounces off resistance more than the other energies and works by *pushing* the resistance out of the person's aura, whereas the softer energies tend to seep through the aura and *transform* the negative charge.)

Slowly, your partner's aura will start to have the same quality of energy and positive charge as your own. Then you won't feel much resistance at all; it will be as if your two auras have almost merged into a single aura, so there will be little that is separate from you to resist you. When that happens, you can touch the top of his head with your hands without losing a significant amount of your field-charge. At this point the channelling should be able to replenish the amount you'll lose without your having to step back. On the other hand, if at any point you feel you need to step back and reestablish the channelling, take the time to do so.

Strange as it may seem, when your two auras become almost equalized, you will probably feel a decrease in the amount of energy flowing, but this is not the same as the slowdown created by the initial resistance from the receiver's negative charge. In this case, because your partner's aura is already charged, there is little energy flow from your aura to his. The energy is still there, but there's little flow. Now is the time to work on specific problems or areas of the body that still need more energy. Hold your hands, while channelling, directly over those problem areas. You can even touch those areas now without collapsing your field-charge, thus concentrating the healing energy directly into the place that needs it most. If there are no specific problems and you are just doing a general revitalization rather than an in-depth overall balancing, this equalization tells you that the channelling is now complete.

THE CHANNELLING

The person who is channelling first stands several feet behind the receiver, who is sitting in a chair. If necessary, you can stand back a little farther, depending upon your own need for space to establish the channelling.

Step 1. First you (the channeller) need to relax, center through receiving your breath, and create the healing mindset.

Step 2. Imagine the white sun eighteen inches to two feet above your head, and develop the energy flow for this method of channelling.

Step 3. When the channelling is established and you feel the energy strongly in your hands, step forward and hold your hands about a foot over the receiver's head, holding them so the palms are halfway facing each other and half pointed down toward the receiver's head. It is easier to feel and maintain the energy when the palms are partially facing each other, for you can feel the energy bouncing back and forth between your hands. At the same time, they need to be partially facing your partner's head so the energy moves that way.

Step 4. Slowly bring your palms closer to the receiver's head. Even though there is just "air" between your hands and his head, you will probably begin to feel some resistance as you get closer. This will decrease with time. If at any point you feel your energy flow decreasing too much, step back, shake your hands, remember the proper mind-set, and reestablish the channelling. It is a good idea to clear yourself like this at least once, and depending upon yourself and the person you are working with, you may need to do this as many as six times or more before your auras are equalized. Remember that there are no trying to's here. All you are doing is opening yourself up to an energy that is already there. You are merely assisting it by being a vehicle for it and directing it through visualization.

Step 5. To help move the energy through your partner, visualize it moving through his head and body, and out his hands and feet. You're not just directing the energy towards his head; you're visualizing it moving through his head and the rest of his body.

Step 6. Do the channelling for fifteen minutes. At the end of that time, your partner should have absorbed enough energy for you to channel with your hands placed directly on top of his head without collapsing your field-charge (although the field-charge may still download a little). Do this for a minute or two. If you prefer, you can wait until you feel your auras are more equalized. Or you can channel while touching his head for ten seconds to see how much downloading occurs, remove your hands and continue to channel until more equalization occurs, and then place your hands on his head again while you continue to channel. Full equalization (not necessary at this point) usually takes approximately a half an hour.

Step 7. When you have placed your hands on the receiver's head and feel ready to move on, you need to step back, shake your hands, and then disconnect your auras, which have become somewhat fused. To do this, hold one palm facing the receiver and one palm facing the ground, and gently move each hand in the direction the palm is facing. You can imagine that you are separating two clouds that have become intermingled. Do this a few feet directly behind the center of his back, then once or twice behind each side of his back, and then a few more times as you step away from him. Most important, keep in mind the *intention* of separating yourself (energy follows thought). (Once when I was working with a woman and there was a knock at the door, I forgot to separate our auras when I went to answer it. The woman had been lying on a table, and when I suddenly walked away from her, she was pulled halfway to a sitting position by the tug of my aura intermingled with and moving away from her own.) If you forget to separate your auras, they will naturally separate over the next few hours. When you do separate auras, your partner will usually feel the shift when he is once again just in his "own space."

Completion. When your auras have been separated, take a few minutes to stretch and relax, and then the receiver will be the channeller. When you have both done the channelling, share your experiences.

It is important to keep in mind that if you feel healing energy in your hands, transference of this energy is taking place whether the other person feels anything or not. I once worked with a very skeptical woman who had a severe hangover. She had taken a couple of aspirins, which hadn't helped her. She decided to allow me to channel for her, in spite of her disbelief that anything could happen, simply because the throbbing in her head hurt enough for her to try anything. I channelled for fifteen minutes, and then I asked her if she had felt anything while I was channelling. She told me she hadn't. But when she stood up she found, to her surprise, that her headache and hangover were completely gone. What the receiver experiences consciously is not necessarily an accurate indicator of what is happening.

4

THE SECOND
METHOD OF
CHANNELLING
HEALING ENERGY

SOURCING FROM THE EARTH

THE PRINCIPLE OF THE SECOND METHOD

In this method of channelling healing energy, we will be using the earth as the energy source. The earth has a healing and mothering quality which promotes a sense of safety and well-being. The color that best generates these qualities is green, so the earth-energy we will be working with mostly will be a green energy, although we will experiment with other colors as well. Green is the basic healing color. It is the color of physical health and growth, and it promotes regeneration. When the body is injured, the aura sends green energy to that area to help in the healing process.

In the first method of channelling we worked with a sunlike energy, so it was natural to source it from above the head. With the second method, since the earth is beneath our feet, it is most natural to pull the energy up through our feet. People who are "airy" types may find the first method easier than this one. Such people often have an emotional resistance to "feeling their feet." On the other hand, "earthy" types of people may find the second method easier. These people may feel a little uneasy sourcing from above; they may feel as if they are getting too lightheaded or unearthly.

The green earth-energy we will be working with doesn't have the sparkle of the white-fire sun-energy; it is smoother and denser, and yet softer (less hard and bouncy) and much more comforting. For example, this green earth-energy works better than the white fire for muscular tension. It penetrates more easily, and its comforting quality helps the muscles to relax and let go. If an organ or a bone needs healing, the earth-energy is most appropriate. However, if an organ is diseased, you might purify it first with white-fire energy, and then give it green earth-energy to help it recuperate and regenerate. This strategy would also work very well for someone with the flu. The key words for this green earth-energy are "security," "health," and "regeneration."

DEVELOPING THE ENERGY

As with the first method, both partners are going to learn the channelling at the same time. So both of you should stand in a relaxed position, with a generous space between you to avoid distractions.

Step 1. When you have taken your position, close your eyes, relax, and center yourself through receiving your breath. Just be aware of yourself standing in the room with a nice-size space around you. When you feel relaxed, imagine that you are standing barefoot in a field of extraordinarily green grass. Really feel the greenness around you. Feel how soothing and healing it is. Then imagine that by relaxing the bottoms of your feet you can soak up into your body the green energy from the grass and the earth. All you have to do is relax, open up the bottoms of your feet, and imagine this green earth-energy seeping into and filling your entire body. Don't try to force the energy to flow. Just allowing the energy to rise up into your body is sufficient to have it happen. Let the energy rise all the way up into your head, and then let it continue to rise, until it reaches the energy center above your head that you used in the first method of channelling. You're not using the sun as an energy source now; you're just letting the earth-energy rise up to it. This may create the feeling that you're standing in a green column of light that goes from your feet to the energy center above your head. If saying "green energy" or "green earth-energy" in your mind helps you to maintain the feeling of the energy, feel free to repeat it to yourself. Essentially, the strength of the earth-energy depends on how open you are to experiencing it and allowing it to move through you. So simply relax and allow yourself to experience the energy flow.

Step 2. When your entire body feels filled with this green earth-energy, hold your hands in front of your body with the palms facing each other. If you just stay relaxed and keep your awareness connected to the source of the energy, within a few minutes you should feel energy in and between your hands. It will feel a little different from the first energy, though, so keep your mind free of expectations of how it should feel. Once you start to feel the energy in your hands, bringing awareness to this feeling (at the same time staying connected to the source of the energy) will increase the strength of the feeling. There may be a tendency to hunch over when using this method of channelling (almost as if you're trying to get closer to the earth, the source of the energy). If you stand straight (not stiff) and relax your back, keeping it open, it will be easier for the energy to rise through your body, all the way up to the energy center above your head. The more space you can make within yourself for the energy, the stronger it will be.

Step 3. When you feel the energy is well established, open your eyes and see if you can maintain the awareness that keeps the energy flowing. See if you can maintain the energy while you are looking at things in the room.

Step 4. When you can channel the energy easily with your eyes open, try using white earth-energy instead of green. Just imagine that you can pull any color energy you want from the earth up through your feet. When you feel established with the white earth-energy, try switching to violet. Then try red. Then blue. Experiment with a few more colors. Notice how different colors feel different when you channel them.

Completion. When you both have finished experimenting with colors, share your experiences with each other. If you should finish before your partner does, do not rush her; give her as much time as she needs.

CHANNELLING THE EARTH-ENERGY TO ANOTHER PERSON

Unlike the sun-energy, the earth-energy does not work with a field-charge, so you don't have to think about your charged auric field collapsing. Although your aura will become charged using this second method of channelling, it will not become overcharged with an excess of energy. Also, since this energy is denser, lower pitched, and less forceful than the sun-energy, it doesn't move as fast and the charge in your aura can't move out as quickly. Therefore, although touching a person's body too quickly with this healing energy will slow down its flow and may even stop it (as the other person's undercharged aura drains off your earth-energy charge), you will not be thrown out of balance, and after stepping back and shaking your hands, you should be able to restart the channelling immediately. Still, to avoid confusion it is best to work slowly through the receiver's aura to her physical body. As with the first method, when you start charging the aura, debris and negative charges may accumulate on your hands, resisting your channelling. If you feel the energy flow slowing down significantly, you need to stop and clear yourself. Just step back, shake your hands to the side, and reestablish the energy flow. Then you can resume channelling. At some point the receiver's aura will become fully charged, and the same kind of equalization that occurred with the first method will take place. At that point, you can go on to more specific work or end the channelling and disconnect your auras (see Step 7, page 27).

THE CHANNELLING

The person who is channelling stands several feet behind the receiver, who is sitting on a chair.

Step 1. First you (the channeller) need to relax, center through receiving your breath, and create the healing mind-set.

Step 2. Imagine that you are standing in a field of extraordinarily green grass, open the bottoms of your feet, and develop the energy flow for this method of channelling. Remember to keep your back open and relaxed. See if you can allow the energy to go all the way up to the energy center above your head.

Step 3. Hold your hands in front of you, and when you feel the energy flow between them, step closer to the receiver and gradually work your way through the denser parts of the aura around her head. When necessary, step back and shake your hands, remember the proper mind-set, and reestablish the channelling.

Step 4. While you are channelling, remember to visualize

the energy moving down from the receiver's head, through her entire body, and out her hands and feet.

Step 5. While you are channelling, try "looking down the energy" into the receiver's body. This means that, since the energy is pervading her body and you are connected to that energy, as you visualize it moving through her, you may be able to "look down the energy" and see where the energy flow is blocked. This is using the energy as an X ray. As you look down the energy, some of you may be able to intuitively *sense* a blockage more easily than you will *see* one. Don't be discouraged if you can't do either yet; it will come with time. If you can see or sense a block, send more energy to that area (without moving your hands from above her head) and see if you can move the block, directing it out one of the extremities. When looking for blocks, you can check the various organs and joints, including the pelvic area. ("Looking down the energy" can also be done with the first method of channelling. I didn't mention it earlier only to avoid overwhelming you with too many possibilities too quickly.) Remember when necessary to step back and shake your hands. Remember, too, that there are no trying to's. You are not creating this energy; it already exists. All you are doing is allowing yourself to feel the energy and be a vehicle for it. The strength of the energy comes primarily from your openness to it.

Step 6. Continue the channelling for ten or fifteen minutes, and then place your hands on the top of your partner's head and continue to channel for a couple of minutes longer.

Step 7. Return your hands to just above your partner's head and channel white earth-energy for a couple of minutes; then switch to violet. (Violet is often a good color to work with because it has a high spiritual vibration.) Continue to experiment with other colors. You can also experiment with having your partner try to guess what color you are channelling. Tell your partner whenever you are about to change to a new color.

Completion. When you are finished, step back, shake your hands, and then disconnect your auras (see Step 7, page 27). Take a few minutes to stretch, and discuss your experiences with the colors. Then change roles so the receiver will be the channeller.

5

THE THIRD
METHOD OF
CHANNELLING
HEALING ENERGY

SOURCING FROM THE
HEART

THE PRINCIPLE OF THE THIRD METHOD

For the third method of channelling healing energy, we use the spiritual heart as the energy source. The fundamental quality of this energy is love. And because everything in the universe radiates some quality of love, we will be able to use this "heart-channelling" to reproduce any healing vibration we are familiar with and channel it through our hands.

Heart-channelling uses an energy that is less dense than the other two healing energies and that has the least quality of force or power. Yet it is as powerful as the others—even more powerful in the situations it is best suited for. Because it is the softest energy it can penetrate the hardest muscle-tension knots. And being such a subtle energy, it penetrates very deeply into a person's being and can release the roots of physical disease: deeply locked emotional and psychic trauma. Sometimes you may want to use one of the other two methods first, to clear out blockages on a denser, more physical level, and then use heart-channelling to create a deeper transformation. I usually recommend this strategy for the longer, in-depth balancings that we will do in the second half of the book.

People who are predominantly emotional or spiritual may take to this way of channelling more easily than people who are more rationally oriented. Most people, though, will be able to learn all three methods, even if they develop a favorite.

There are many ways to create a source for this third method of channelling. The most direct way is simply to create within yourself a state of unconditional love for the person you are working with. That love would be the energy source for the channelling. And because this does not take your mind away from what is happening in the present moment, it enables you to be more connected to your partner and more aware of what is happening inside him. Also, because using it teaches you how to experience people through unconditional love, it tends to foster in the channeller more personal and spiritual growth than the other methods. For these reasons, this way of sourcing from the heart is preferable, but each person should use the method that works best for her. (It may help to reread the section on unconditional love, page 12.)

If you are religious or spiritually oriented, you could imagine that you are in God's presence, or are feeling divine love, or the love of a saint or spiritual leader. As the feeling grows in your heart, you can allow its energy to spread to your hands, so you can channel it for the other person.

If you are not religious in nature, you could remember the moment in your life when you felt the most happiness, ecstasy, or love (remember Exercise 1, page 5). You could use the memory of that feeling to generate a heart-channelling that you can share with the other person in the present. This could also be done using a fantasy as your source, or by simply imagining the deepest quality of love you think is possible for you to feel. As you imagine it, you will feel it.

If you are a parent, you could use your love for your children as a source. You might even try to perceive the child within the adult you are channelling for, to help bring out those nurturing, loving feelings within yourself.

There are also innumerable less obvious sources. Do you love the smell of roses? You could imagine yourself filled with the smell and essence of roses. You could either channel the love you feel for roses or think of the aroma as a particular quality of love that a rose gives off, and then simply let that love, the love from the rose itself, go through you, just as you let the earth-energy go through you. But now, instead of going through your feet, the love from the rose moves through your heart. Then you are actually *channelling roses*. Similarly, you could channel any flower or plant, or even any crystal energy whose healing properties would be appropriate for a particular situation. (With crystals, you just remember the way that crystal's energy feels—its particular quality of love—and let it move through your heart and hands.) In fact, with this method *you can draw on any quality of love you perceive and become a channel for it to pass through your heart and hands*.

Just as with the first two methods, there are no trying to's here. This heart-energy already exists; you don't have to create it. How well it comes through depends entirely upon how willing you are to experience it. The heart-energy will feel much finer and softer in your hands than the first two energies. It may have a certain sparkle to it, but if it does, it will be a much softer sparkle than the sun-energy's. This heart-energy is extremely gentle. In the *Tao Te Ching* it says:

> The softest thing in the universe
> Overcomes the hardest thing in the universe.

That without substance
Can enter where there is no room. *

The key words for this heart-energy are "unconditional love."

DEVELOPING THE ENERGY

As with the first two methods, both partners will learn the channelling at the same time.

Step 1. Close your eyes, relax, forget about your partner, and center yourself through receiving your breath. Just be aware of yourself standing in the room with a comfortable space around you. Then choose whichever method appeals to you to develop this heart-energy. If you are going to use unconditional love, imagine that there is someone (other than your partner†) in front of you for whom you feel this unconditional love. Whatever source you are using to connect yourself to the heart-energy of this channelling, allow yourself to experience as much of that love as you can. Fill yourself with this love. Let yourself surrender to it completely. With heart-energy it is not important to be aware of your feet or the energy center above your head. With this method you are mainly using your feelings, and it will help to experience them in the area of your heart. It may also help to say the word "love" in your mind or to visualize a color for the energy or feelings, or to receive your breath in your heart. Use whatever works for you.

---

*From Verse 43, *Tao Te Ching*, by Lao Tsu. Translated by Gia-Fu Feng and Jane English (New York: Vintage, 1972).

†The reason for not using your partner at this point is that he will telepathically receive the channelling, disrupting his own practice of the exercise. Later, when you are channelling for each other, your partner should be the focus of the love.

Step 2. When you feel yourself smiling inside with all the love that is pouring through you, hold your hands in front of you and feel the love energy in your hands. Remember, this energy will feel soft. Also remember that you don't have to make the energy go to your hands; you just have to allow yourself to feel it going there. If you find yourself hunching over, stand up straighter and let your back relax and open up so the heart area of your body is more open. When you feel the energy in your hands, bringing awareness to this feeling (at the same time staying connected to the source of the energy) will increase its strength.

Step 3. When you feel the heart-energy is well established, open your eyes and see if you can maintain the awareness that keeps the energy flowing. See if you can maintain the energy while you are looking at things in the room.

Completion. When you can channel the energy easily with your eyes open, you may stop. When you have both stopped, share your experiences with each other. If you finish before your partner does, do not rush him; give him as much time as he needs.

CHANNELLING THE HEART-ENERGY TO ANOTHER PERSON

The heart-energy does not use any kind of field-charge whatsoever. Because this energy is so much more subtle than the other two, it tends to seep into the debris and transform it rather than push against it. So your partner's aura, in general, will be less resistant to your channelling with this method. Still, if at any point you lose the channelling, step back, shake your hands, and recenter. As with the other methods, the receiver's aura will eventually become fully charged, and an equalization will result. At that point, you can go on to work on specific areas or end the channelling and disconnect your auras (see Step 7, page 27).

THE CHANNELLING

The person who is channelling stands several feet behind the receiver, who is sitting in a chair.

Step 1. First you (the channeller) need to relax, center through receiving your breath, and create the healing mind-set.

Step 2. Use whatever method you have chosen to generate the heart-energy.

Step 3. When you feel the energy in your hands, step closer and begin the channelling. Gradually work your way through the denser parts of the aura around the receiver's head. Remember that there are no trying to's; you only have to open up or surrender to the energy that is already there.

Step 4. While you are channelling, remember to visualize the energy moving through your partner's body and out his hands and feet. As you do this, "look down the energy" and actually see it go through his body. Check the organs, joints, and the pelvic area for blockages. If you become aware of a block, direct more energy to it by visualizing your heart-energy either washing it away, melting it, slipping underneath it and prying it loose, or just dissolving it. If any debris comes loose from the block, you can send it out one of the extremities. Remember to step back and shake your hands when necessary.

Step 5. Do the channelling for fifteen minutes, and then place your hands on the top of your partner's head and continue to channel for a couple of minutes longer.

Completion. When you are finished, step back, shake your hands, and then disconnect your auras (see Step 7, page 27). Take a few minutes to stretch, and then the receiver will be the channeller. Share your experiences when you are both done.

6

COLORS

Every color has its own unique healing properties. When working with a particular color, visualize as clear a color as you can. Muddy colors lack energy and will not promote much healing. You can use the second method of channelling healing energy to channel any color. Just imagine that the earth is filled with whatever color you need, and feel that color come up through your feet. (The first method of channelling can be used for most colors, but I would advise against using red, which does not work well with the energy centers involved in this method. Orange, though, would be fine.)

People who can see auras detect many colors in every person's aura. Usually one or two colors predominate, which indicates something about the person. The color of her aura, though, has nothing to do with what color would be best for you to channel for her. Also, while each color and method of channelling help certain kinds of situations best, the three methods of channelling you have learned can each, with any color, be used for all situations.

Here is a description of the properties, uses, and significance of the healing colors:

Red is the color of physical energy. It is used to energize. Care must be taken with this color, though, as it is easy to overenergize, causing restlessness. It can be very good for a sluggish liver. When a person releases red energy while you are working on him, it usually represents anger, but this is very different from channelling red as a healing energy. Sometimes people have red as the predominant color in their aura. This has nothing to do with anger and just connotes a general physical strength and vibrancy. Such people are often warm and affectionate individuals.

Orange is the color of emotional happiness. This color would be very good for a person who needs more laughter in her life. It is a good color for the bladder and the front of the hips. Sometimes a cloudy orange is seen in an aura where there is some kind of physical irritation. A clear orange would represent happiness.

Green is the basic color of physical healing. It promotes growth, health, security, and regeneration. It also represents individualism and the ego. The predominant color of most auras is green because most people spend the greatest part of their time occupied with issues related to the third chakra, which is mostly green (see page 69). When concentrations of green are found in a particular area, it indicates that healing is taking place there.

Yellow is the color of the intellect. If a person's thinking is confused, yellow would be a good color for him. People who are intellectual or who make their living using their minds often have a lot of yellow in their auras, especially in the area of the head. It is a good color for the kidneys and can be used as a general toner for the system.

Pink is the color of unconditional emotional love. It combines white unconditional spiritual love (from the higher chakras) with red emotion (from the lower chakras). Pink would nourish a person who needs a lot of love and nurturing or who has trouble giving love. Channel it especially into the second chakra (just above the pubic bone) and the heart chakra. This color is not generally used for physical healing. A predominantly pink aura represents a modest, perhaps quiet, but loving individual. It may also represent a large capacity for devotion.

Gold has a quality of permanence that no other color has. If someone has broken a bone, for instance, lay down lines of gold energy, reconnecting the halves of the break to create a structure for the healing, and then surround the whole area with green light for general physical healing. Gold is the color for restructuring. It is also very spiritual; like white, it represents unconditional spiritual love. Gold auras are rare.

Blue is the color of peace. If someone is disturbed, worried, overexcited, or angry, blue would help to restore calm and peacefulness. The same principle would apply to something like an upset stomach. Blue is very soothing and quieting. It can be used for most situations as a general healing color and is especially good for those that require rest and recuperation. If a person's nerves are too excited or exhausted, channelling blue (and then white) into her spleen chakra, which is involved with nerve balance, would be helpful (see page 70). It is sometimes found as the predominant color of a person's aura, indicating a spiritually inclined, peace-loving individual. Light blue would indicate, in addition, an idealistic nature.

Purple is a mixture of blue and red. In a person's aura it represents spirituality mixed with passion. Sometimes it represents wisdom, which is spiritual (blue) knowledge gained through worldly (red) experience. People who have a lot of anger, which is "negative" red energy, might benefit from this color. Instead of quieting the anger as blue would do, the purple would seep into or be absorbed by the negative red energy (due to the red within the purple), penetrating it and transforming it. Purple might also prove useful for an individual who has a lot of worldly experience that has not yet developed into wisdom.

Violet represents spiritual meditation. It also stimulates psychic awareness. It is used more for general spiritual or emotional healing than for physical healing. Usually violet is found in significant amounts in a person's aura only when he has reached an advanced level in his spiritual growth.

White has all colors in it, including all the healing colors, so it can be used for any kind of healing. It also represents purity, protection, and unconditional spiritual love. If you feel threatened by a situation and you imagine yourself surrounded by a cocoon of white light, it will help to protect you. White represents a very high degree of spirituality. Predominantly white auras are very rare.

Experiment with different colors. Ask your partner (and others you practice with) how she feels when you channel various colors. If you begin to see colors in people's auras, remember that the clearness of the color can tell you as much about the person as the particular color you find.

7

THE ILLUSION
OF PICKING UP
OTHER PEOPLE'S
"STUFF"

The issue of "picking up other people's Stuff"* is important, and it will crop up over and over again in any future studies you pursue concerning healing. There are many myths and fears surrounding this issue, but the unchanging truth is really very simple: *You cannot pick up anyone else's Stuff; the only Stuff you can have is your own.*

Many people misguidedly believe that if they are not careful when they release negative charges from someone they are working with, they will pick up this Stuff and absorb it into

*The word "Stuff" is commonly used by healers, meditators, and spiritual seekers to describe all our various forms of "negative" energy: anger, fear, self-pity, general toxicity, destructive or limiting beliefs and attitudes, and so on. The idea that this is all just Stuff reminds us that it is not part of who we really are and that these experiences are not actually negative; they are simply various forms of our resistance to experiencing "the Light." They represent our mental/emotional/physical/spiritual unclearness, the general Stuff of the human condition that we are here to experience and transform.

themselves. Many of these people also fear that they may pick up someone else's headache, exhaustion, or even disease. They feel vulnerable because of the openness of the state they are in when they are chanelling (or massaging); and hence they have come up with methods for "protecting" themselves.

As common as these beliefs are, they have no validity whatsoever. Here is an example of the experiences that give rise to these myths: Let's say I am doing a healing session with someone who is grieving. If I have a lot of suppressed or unresolved grief within myself, then becoming aware of the receiver's grief may trigger and bring to the surface my own. At the end of the session, I may feel sad and think that I have picked up the other person's grief, but this is a misperception; the only grief I have—or can ever experience—is my own.

This process is very similar to watching a movie. If it is a sad film, it may make us feel sad through our identification with the characters. But for most of us, this sadness is gone by the time we're out in the parking lot. Yet what about those few people who end up feeling sad all the rest of the night and perhaps even for days afterwards? Have they picked up this sadness from the movie? It should be pretty obvious that they have some personal Stuff about sadness that the movie has brought to the surface. (And the more powerful the movie, the more people it is able to trigger in this way.)

What happens when you watch a person release sadness during a healing session is not very different from watching a film character go through some sad experience. And the deeper, more powerful the emotion the receiver is releasing, the deeper you may be triggered, too. It is important to re-member that whatever you are experiencing emotionally is just your own emotional response—you are not picking up any-thing from the other person. Although a certain person may always trigger a particular feeling or resistance in you that makes it hard for you to stay clear (of "negative" feelings), this unclarity is your own Stuff triggered but not caused by the other person. Whatever you resist (or react to) in other people is always what you resist and are afraid of experiencing within yourself. (The converse is also true: whatever you resist within yourself you will resist in other people.) You are responsible for your own state of beingness; *the only Stuff you can ever have is your own*.

Yet even when our own emotions are triggered by the other person, what really gets us stuck during a channelling is our reaction to these emotions. When we resist or react to our own triggered emotions we become caught up in a struggle with ourselves, blocking energy flow and getting ourselves stuck.*

Therefore, the key to staying clear during a channelling is to cultivate towards yourself and the other person an attitude of *conscious acceptance and nonreaction*. This means that if an emotion is coming up (in you or the other person), you don't resist the feeling, push it away, identify with it, or feed it; you simply accept the feeling and allow it to be there. You stay detached and give it some space. Then you are simply observing whatever emotion comes up, instead of getting caught up in it and struggling with it (and therefore being controlled by it). Then it just passes through like the weather, like passing thoughts, and leaves you in a clear place. In

---

*It is also possible, without getting stuck, to consciously "pattern" or "mirror" to some degree in your own body what the other person is releasing, or even still holding. (I do this frequently myself.) It enables you to feel in your own body what is stuck or being released by the other person. Patterning does not involve triggering your own Stuff nor taking on the other person's Stuff. It's putting your foot temporarily into someone else's shoe to understand how it feels. Unless some of your own Stuff is triggered, you can always take your foot out. Sometimes a channeller patterns unconsciously. If you do, when the other person becomes clear, you will find yourself clear as well. Patterning is a wonderful tool. And it doesn't change the bottom line: the only Stuff you ever have is your own.

general, this is simply learning to *be* with yourself and others, instead of *doing* things to resist or react to what is happening.

"Conscious acceptance and nonreaction" is really the same as the "proper mind-set" described in Chapter 2. To accept someone and allow them to be as they are, you also need to allow yourself to be as you are. Otherwise, every time something in you is triggered and you resist it (a form of negating yourself), you will resist the person who is triggering you as well. To genuinely feel unconditional love for someone else, you also need to feel unconditional love for yourself. This is one of the most wonderful aspects of learning how to heal other people: you learn to heal yourself. (At the very least, you find out where you are stuck.)

The process of becoming stuck by resisting someone else's feelings (really your own) is not restricted to healing situations. It happens all the time in everyday life. The depressed friend who "got me down" is not really the cause of my feeling bad. I depress myself with my own resistance and with whatever triggered feelings I had suppressed. What happens during a channelling session is just an intensification of what happens all the time in everyday life. The consequences of resistance are more apparent, but the same rules apply.

There is a strange irony concerning this issue. Although you cannot pick up anyone else's Stuff, if you fear and believe strongly enough that you can, then it is possible you will re-create the other person's condition within yourself. You do have this power, for energy follows thought, so you tend to become what you fear/resist the most. But if this happens, the other person will not have given you this condition; you will have created it for yourself out of your own resistance and fear. Again: all you will have is your own Stuff.

If your fears of picking up other people's Stuff are still very strong, then either you should use your channelling sessions as a way of contacting and transforming these fears, or you should not be channelling for others at this time; work instead on yourself.

In Part II you will learn how to clear your own aura after doing an in-depth balancing. But remember, this is not to clear out the Stuff you've picked up from the other person; it's to clear out your own Stuff that has been triggered and brought to the surface by your resistance during the channelling.

8

LOOSE
ENDS

Working on Yourself. Any of the methods for channelling healing energy can be used on yourself. As you have probably noticed by now, you feel better after channelling for someone else. Channelling healing energy is self-healing and purifies your own aura. If you want to work on specific problems in yourself, establish a channelling and then visualize the energy going to the problem area, opening it up, dissolving the blockage, and washing it out through one of your extremities. Or visualize any other image that works for you. If holding your hands in front of you and feeling the healing energy in them helps you to maintain the energy flow, you can do that too. You can even establish the healing energy in your hands and then channel with your hands into the problem area.

Expectations. You shouldn't be discouraged if at first you don't experience everything described here. Babies are very aware of etheric energy, but because Western society pays most attention to sexual and emotional energy, we have forgotten how to recognize what we once knew. So give yourself time. Expectations will eventually get you caught up with trying to's, which will block energy flow and lead to frustration. Whenever this happens, *stop*, step back, reestablish the proper mind-set, and then resume the channelling. In the end, this will shorten the amount of time needed for the healing session and will make it easier and more enjoyable.

Touching When Channelling. The problem with touching someone while channelling for them is that if you are working with a field-charge, the energy may be transferred too quickly, disrupting your energy field and aura. As I explained earlier, this is most likely to happen during the first (sun-energy) method of channelling. In general, there are two possible solutions. The first is the one I've already recommended: Clear the aura and problem area first without touching it, and then touch the body directly. Another approach is to touch the person *before* you start channelling: at this point there is no field-charge to create a significant difference in energy between your aura and hers. Now when you begin to channel, both of your auras will increase in energy at a close enough rate that you won't experience the breakdown of your field-charge. Many people prefer to use this method for hands-on channelling, whereas others find it more difficult to first establish the channelling while they are touching the other person. Choose the method that works best for you.

Touching the other person when channelling is most important when dealing with muscle knots or various kinds of traumatized tissue, for in these situations the tension is locked inside or beneath tissue that has become hardened. Touching the tight or hardened area while channelling helps to prevent the healing energy from simply bouncing off the tissue knot.

Looking Down the Energy. If you can't do this yet, be patient; you will be able to in time. If you can't actually see energy going into the receiver, it is still important to visualize it doing so, and in either case it is important to see it (actually or imaginatively) going throughout her body, or with specific problems, into the heart of the problem area. Energy follows thought. Where you think it, there it will move.

Visualization. A simple way of getting the healing energy into the core of a specific problem area is to see or visualize a healthy place underneath or inside the problem, even if it is very tiny and under many layers of tension or disease. Visualize that healthy place receiving the healing energy and growing, until it fills the whole area that had the problem. You can also instruct the receiver to spend a few minutes each day visualizing the problem the way she wants it resolved, in its healthy state, before going to bed. Since energy follows thought, her visualization of health helps to create it.

EXERCISE 3: SORE SPOTS

For this exercise, simply take turns channelling into a sore spot on your partner's body. First try establishing the channelling and clearing the aura in the area around the sore spot before touching it. Once you touch it, keep channelling until you feel it relax. Then put your hands directly on another sore spot, and while you are touching the body, establish the channelling. When you touch the sore spot, press down just enough to feel the tension. Be aware of the healing energy in your fingertips. As you channel, imagine a healthy place inside or underneath the tension and visualize that clear spot receiving the healing energy and growing, spreading through the tension and melting it. Keep channelling until the sore spot relaxes. Use any method of channelling you prefer. Feel free to experiment with colors.

EXERCISE 4: CHANNELLING FROM A DISTANCE

Surprising as it may seem, healing energy can be channelled to people in need even if they are not present. The other person could be in China—or even on the moon—and your healing energy could still reach him.

There are various ways to channel from a distance. I will describe two possible methods here. If any other method works for you, use it.

The best way to practice this exercise is with the receiver and channeller in separate rooms. The channeller closes her eyes, but it is preferable for the receiver to keep his eyes open. (If the receiver's eyes are closed, there may be a tendency to reach out towards the channeller with the aura or consciousness, but the channeller should have to find the receiver without any help.) Each of you can try one of the channelling-from-a-distance methods explained below. Wait until you both have had a chance to channel before sharing your experiences. Then, if you like, repeat it trying the other method.

For the first method, begin by visualizing your partner in your mind. As you do this, try to feel his essence or presence. Try to see and feel him vividly enough to give you the sense that you are actually present with him. It may help to mentally call his name. On some level this tends to attract the receiver's attention and turn him towards you. Then go into the third method of channelling healing energy (sourcing from the heart), and feel your unconditional love go out towards and touch your partner (just as you did in the third part of Exercise 2, on page 13). If there is a specific problem area, feel your love touch him in that place. Remember, energy follows thought.

For the second method, either imagine that something in you can simply reach out through the top of your head and find your partner or imagine a tube of light going from the top of your head to the top of your partner's. (This will be utilizing the crown chakra, which sits on the top of your head.) Once you have felt contact, realize that by whatever method you reached out to touch your partner you can reach out with healing energy and touch him. Maintaining your sense of the connection with your partner, go into the third method of channelling and reach out with your heart-energy, right through the top of your head, touching your partner with it. If there is a specific problem area, feel your energy touch him in that place.

II

CREATING
AN IN-DEPTH
AURA
BALANCING

9

MODELS
OF THE
HUMAN
BODY

Acupuncture introduced the West to a new concept of medicine. Yet Western science, for all its advancement, cannot explain why acupuncture works. The acupuncturists try to explain to the scientists that it works on the body's "energy system" through access points on the body's "meridians"—invisible energy lines that run throughout the body. But Western scientists keep looking for an explanation that fits their own model of how the body works. They cannot imagine that the world can be effectively explained by a model other than their own. These scientists are victims of a fundamental misperception: they believe that their own model for describing reality is actually reality itself. (See Appendix B: "An Alternative Theory of Disease.")

The human body can be interpreted through many different models, and treatments based on some of them provide good reproducible results. Although scientists sometimes learn to translate some of the findings from other models, like acupuncture, into their own model, the result is a bit like translating Chinese into English—something essential is lost in the process. Of course, something is gained too, and the Western model expands as a result of the new translation. But often what is lost in translation is the context that provides the delicate understanding necessary to the successful use of the new information.*

If we truly want to learn what these other models have to offer, we need to learn them from their own points of view. Each of the systems I will describe here presents a model of the human body. Each is a complete science unto itself, and each provides information that will be valuable to us when we work with channelling healing energy.

FIVE SUCCESSFUL MODELS

WESTERN MEDICINE

Western medicine deals with the body in almost exclusively physical terms. It takes little account of the mind, or anything else it cannot measure directly. Its map of the body is a physical map that outlines where the various organs, muscles, nerves, and cellular structures lie and describes how these work together chemically. Western medicine's strength is its ability to repair these parts by operating on them. Its major weakness is its perception of symptoms of disease as equivalent to the disease itself. Therefore it uses drugs to suppress symptoms, leaving the real cause of the disease rooted in the body where

---

*For instance, since Western medicine is geared towards suppressing disease symptoms, it would translate acupuncture or the Japanese healing art of Jin Shin Jyutsu into another means towards that end. Yet these healing arts are not oriented towards suppressing symptoms at all; their purpose is to create harmony within the human being (through balancing the body), in the belief that a body in harmony heals itself.

it will continue to grow (inward now instead of outward) and likely show up as a greater problem later on. In addition, the weakening effect of the drugs on the body as a whole (virtually all drugs have negative side effects) cause the real problem to grow worse even faster. * Treating symptoms as the disease also forces Western medicine to view the body compartmentally. For weakness in the eyes, only the eyes are examined, even though their weakness may be only a symptom of problems elsewhere in the body. The root problem will continue to worsen and to create other symptoms if it remains unnoticed and untreated. Also, because Western medicine concentrates on suppressing symptoms, it has not developed a deep enough understanding of the body to actually heal it. Doctors can advise patients to rest, give them a pill, or remove one of their parts, but they have little knowledge of how to strengthen and balance the system. Yet in spite of its limitations, the Western medical model is very successful at what it does best: operating on diseased body parts. And the field of genetic engineering will open new areas in which Western medicine will prove very effective.

PSYCHOTHERAPY

Psychotherapy views the body in terms of its connection to the mind. According to this model many diseases are caused by emotional problems or attitudes, which are expressed symbolically as diseases or other problems in the physical body. An example of this mind-body connection is a client who had cancer in his back, which was caused by the grief he was holding in after his best friend slept with his wife. Although

---

*An example of this was a client of mine who had suffered from asthma for twelve years. He had been on medication to suppress the asthma, and after twelve years the asthma disappeared. But as soon as it disappeared he developed diabetes.

he wasn't conscious of the link between his cancer and his grief, he stated over and over again: "I felt like my friend stabbed me in the back."

ACUPUNCTURE

Acupuncture's model presents the body as governed by a nonphysical (actually, less physical) *energy system*. This energy system functions as a higher-level nervous system that controls and feeds both the physical nervous system and all the physical functions and activities of the body. The body's energy system is also the link between mind and body, between the (nonphysical) energy phenomena of thought and emotion and the physical body.

Acupuncture treats the physical body by working on the body's energy system. According to this model, physical problems are external symptoms of blockages that *existed in the body's energy system* prior to their physical appearance in specific parts of the body. Knowledge of this energy system enables an acupuncturist to discover and clear the energy block before it manifests itself as a physical problem.

In acupuncture, the body's energy system is composed of meridians, which are energy lines that run throughout the body. There are devices that can locate and measure acupuncture points—energized points along the meridian lines. Each major organ is governed by a meridian; there are fourteen major (and fifty-seven minor) meridians altogether. Diseases develop when these lines of energy become blocked or unbalanced. Needles inserted into acupuncture points can rebalance the meridians and thus the body's entire energy system. It is even possible to anesthetize parts of the body, making operations possible without the use of drugs. Unfortunately, many contemporary acupuncturists use a Western model of acupuncture ("textbook acupuncture") and do not have the effectiveness of those who are traditionally trained. One of the reasons for this Westernization is that it takes many years to develop the traditional understanding of and attunement to the body.

JIN SHIN JYUTSU

This is a little-known but very powerful Japanese healing art which, like acupuncture, works by helping energy to flow through the body. (I use Jin Shin Jyutsu a lot in my own healing practice.) Here, disease is a symptom of mental, emotional, or physical stress-created blockages in the energy pathways of the body's energy system. The model or energy map of the body is loosely similar to but much more complex than acupuncture's meridian map. Yet Jin Shin is very simple to practice (there are only 26 points, called "safety energy locks," on each side of the body, compared to traditional acupuncture's 309), and it is designed for people to easily use on themselves. *

Jin Shin Jyutsu utilizes a universal energy that flows throughout the body, making use of what is flowing through the practitioner's hands to recharge the receiver's energy in blocked areas. The healing energy can be concentrated in different parts of the energy system (to help weak body functions and related emotions) by placing the hands on the twenty-six points in various combinations. The recharged energy is then able to release the stress-created blockages in the energy pathways, restoring harmony to the system. Body, mind, emotion, and spirit are brought back into balance (in rhythm with the universe). Jin Shin Jyutsu can be practiced at almost any time, even while watching television. It works right through cloth-

*Books on Jin Shin Jyutsu are hard to find. Mary Burmeister, the recognized world authority on this art, has published several simple self-help books for people who have not had the opportunity to take her more comprehensive workshops. For information about obtaining these books, write to Jin Shin Jyutsu, Inc., 8719 E. San Alberto, Scottsdale, AZ 85258.

ing, and will even work through a plaster cast. The Jin Shin Jyutsu model also maps out the major organ–emotion relationships; for instance, fear affects the bladder and kidneys, and weakness in these organs makes a person more susceptible to fear. (Traditional acupuncture also makes use of these body-emotion connections, and Western medicine is now discovering that certain diseases have "emotional profiles.") I will outline these connections in the next chapter.

YOGIC CHAKRA SYSTEM

Chakra is a Sanskrit word for "wheel." The chakras are energy centers in the body's energy system that looked like glowing wheels (one to several inches in diameter, with spokes) to the Indian yogis who discovered them. Each chakra has its own functions much as each organ does; in a sense, they are "energy-organs." And just as the digestive organs make up a digestive system, the chakras all work together and make up a chakra system. Traditionally there are seven major chakras and many minor ones (see illustration on page 68). The major chakras lie in a vertical line between the spine and the front of the body, and radiate out both the back and front of the body. Although I have not come across any information that completely ties together the chakra system, the acupuncture meridian system, and the Jin Shin Jyutsu energy map, they are each different aspects of one body energy system, working together. It is no coincidence that the most important energy lines in both acupuncture and Jin Shin Jyutsu lie on the spine and the center front of the body, overlaying the major chakras.

For yogis, the most important part of the chakra system is the "kundalini energy" which flows up the spine. The kundalini energy both feeds the chakras and is fed by them. It also feeds the nerves. The kundalini is often called the "sleeping serpent," because in ordinary people its more powerful aspects are in an inactive state, lying dormant at the base of the spine.

Through meditation and other energy techniques, this sleeping energy can be awakened and made to travel up the spine, intensely charging the chakras, expanding spiritual awareness and bestowing psychic powers, until it pours out the top of the head, through the crown chakra. The kundalini has three aspects. One goes straight up the spine, and the other two weave back and forth across the spine, like serpents. This is the origin of the caduceus—the symbol of two serpents winding up a staff, which is the traditional emblem of a physician or healer. (In classical times the caduceus was a symbol worn by sacred or holy people, many of whom were actively working with this energy.) The kundalini is also known as the "serpent fire," because of the firelike quality of its energy when deeply awakened.

Although utilizing healing energy activates the kundalini a little (in yourself as well as the person you are working with), for the in-depth aura balancing we will not work directly with our kundalini "fire." The chakras will be the main focus of our attention. Since the chakras are energy centers, they are natural areas to use for the transference of healing energy.

HOMEOPATHY

Homeopathy is a branch of medicine that is experiencing a resurgence in the United States. It was once very popular here and has been popular in Europe where natural medicine is more widely used. (In England, the royal family has been under homeopathic care since the 1930s.) Homeopathy declined in the United States at the turn of the century for mostly political reasons. Most homeopathy is practiced here today by naturopathic doctors. With spiralling medical costs, many lay-people are also teaching themselves how to use homeopathy for first aid and illness, and homeopathic study groups are cropping up around the country.

The basic principle of homeopathy is that like cures like. An example would be curing a poison ivy outbreak with a remedy created from poison ivy. This remedy could also be used to cure other similar skin conditions. Unlike vaccinations, however, which inject actual dead or weakened germs into the body, a homeopathic remedy made from poison ivy will not, in its final form, contain any actual poison ivy. In the making of the remedy, the solution or powder of poison ivy is repeatedly energized and diluted. By the time it is finished, it has been so diluted that there are no more molecules of poison ivy left. But the subtle essence of the poison ivy remains. In a sense, the *aura* of the poison ivy plant is imprinted onto the remedy. And this energy imprint of the poison ivy works on the energy system of the body receiving it.

There are several possible explanations of how homeopathic remedies work. Here's one: since the remedy contains "subtle poison ivy," it will stimulate the body's immune response to poison ivy on a subtle but deep level. This helps the body to overcome the actual poison ivy symptoms on a physical level. (Sometimes this will actually make the symptoms worsen for a very short time—a positive sign that the remedy is working.)

These remedies are very effective. Without drugs, they can cure disease conditions, sometimes miraculously fast, and strengthen the body in the process without causing side effects.

The homeopathic principle of using like to cure like can be used with energy channelling when, intuitively, the channeller feels that the only way a particular emotion will be released is by amplifying it and forcing it to the surface. For example, red might be channelled into an area that is holding anger as a way to force the anger to emerge and release. When channelling, this approach should be a last resort, but it is an option that will help in certain circumstances.

10

AN ECLECTIC BODY

When we do the in-depth balancing, we will make use of
information and awareness gained from all the systems of healing outlined in Chapter 9. We will be working with an "eclectic
body," ranging from spleens and livers to chakras, energy flow,
and mind-body connections.

THE CHAKRA SYSTEM

The chakra system is a major component of the eclectic
body. Much of the in-depth balancing involves working with
the chakra system. The illustration on the following page shows
the most important chakras. Traditionally the major chakras
are those numbered one through seven.

First Chakra. This is the root chakra, also called the survival chakra. It is located at the bottom of the spine. Since its

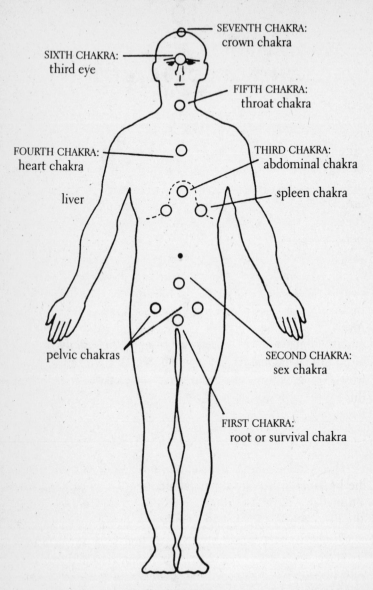

EIGHTH CHAKRA

SEVENTH CHAKRA:
crown chakra

SIXTH CHAKRA:
third eye

FIFTH CHAKRA:
throat chakra

FOURTH CHAKRA:
heart chakra

THIRD CHAKRA:
abdominal chakra

liver

spleen chakra

pelvic chakras

SECOND CHAKRA:
sex chakra

FIRST CHAKRA:
root or survival chakra

THE CHAKRAS

primary function is to ensure survival, survival fears show up here. This chakra affects the adrenals, kidneys, and bladder, which are also weakened by fear. If you feel safe and secure, this chakra will be clear. Predominant colors: reds.

Second Chakra. Although this is called the sex chakra, it is actively involved in all forms of intimacy and interpersonal emotions and strongly affects your sense of emotional well-being. Emotional love has its roots here. It is located in the area just above the pubic bone. If a person feels sexually aroused, a lot of energy moves to and radiates from this chakra. It is also involved in the reproductive system. If there are blocks here, they may eventually affect the sexual organs and the general hip area. Predominant colors: oranges and reds.

Third Chakra. This is the abdominal chakra. It is located in the area of the solar plexus. This chakra influences the intellect as well as self-protection, personal will, and physical power and control. This involves all forms of competing, and hence also frustration and anger. If you are competitive, angry, frustrated, or self-protective, you will have a lot of tension in this area. This tension may eventually show up in the stomach, liver, gallbladder, or spleen, all of which work closely with this chakra. Predominant colors: greens and yellows.

Fourth Chakra. This is the heart chakra. It is located near the heart, in the center of the chest. It is the seat of unconditional spiritual love. (Unconditional *emotional* love is the emotional energy of the second chakra rising up to and resonating with the unconditional spiritual love of the fourth chakra.) When this chakra opens, its energy rises and resonates with the higher chakras. When it is blocked, self-alienation and self-hatred from deep emotional trauma will be found here. These emotions adversely affect the immune system, so opening the heart chakra strengthens the immune system both by releasing these emotions and by its beneficial effect on the thymus, which is located near it. This chakra is the first to deal with the spiritual aspects of our Self; the first three all deal with physical survival in some form. Most people keep the largest part of their awareness in their first three chakras. The heart chakra represents the level of awareness the human race is presently trying to evolve into. Predominant colors: gold, white, pink, raspberry.

Fifth Chakra. This is the throat chakra. It is located at the bottom of the throat. It controls creativity, communication, and clairaudience (psychic hearing), and can signify purity. People who block their creativity or communication will be blocked here. The throat chakra affects the thyroid and is therefore—along with the adrenals and liver—vital for energy production and metabolism. Predominant colors: white, silver, blues.

Sixth Chakra. This is the third eye. It is located between the eyebrows and affects the pituitary and pineal glands. This chakra controls clairvoyance and psychic perception. It is considered the doorway to eternity. Predominant colors: blues, purples, indigos, white.

Seventh Chakra. This is the crown chakra. It is located at the center-top of the head. (When it is fully open it covers the whole top of the head, like a crown.) This is usually considered the highest chakra. It connects you to God or All That Is. It is also used for telepathic healing. The radiance of this chakra formed the halo that was reported to be visible around Jesus' head. This is where the soul enters the body. Predominant colors: white, violet, or a rainbow effect.

* * *

Eighth Chakra. There is no common name for this chakra. Many systems don't include it because it is not located in the body, although it is in the aura. It is located eighteen inches to two feet above the head. It works with the third eye and other higher chakras to connect you to your higher Self and is considered the intersection point between the body's aura and the soul's energy. Because so much energy flows through the eighth chakra, it is a good source for healing energy. It also governs intuitive knowledge. When you know something is going to happen but you don't know how you know it, that soul-awareness information comes from your eighth chakra. (There is no specific color for this chakra.)

Spleen Chakra. The spleen chakra is located at the bottom of the rib cage on the lefthand side. (There are some systems that leave out the sex chakra and use the spleen as the second chakra for fear that conscious work with the sex chakra will overstimulate and distract the yogi, who is supposed to keep his mind on spiritual matters.) The spleen chakra absorbs energy from the sun and feeds it to the aura, influencing vitality and balancing the nervous system. It interacts with the adrenals, liver, and third chakra. People who suffer from allergies or nervousness usually need help in their spleen chakra. The spleen strengthens the immune system. Predominant color: white.

Liver. The liver is not usually considered a chakra, but we will be working with it as if it were one because energy is usually blocked there, and the liver works closely with the spleen and ties into the third chakra. It is located at the bottom of the rib cage on the right. The liver controls the eyes and body chemistry, so it needs help when a person has weak eyes or suffers from allergies, hypoglycemia, or exhaustion. On an emotional level, the liver stores frustration and anger. (When the anger is deep and bitter, it is usually held in the gall-bladder.) Red is a good color for a sluggish liver or for bringing anger stored in the liver to the surface. Purple is more effective for transforming anger.

Pelvic Chakras. Although the pelvic chakras are not traditionally considered part of the major chakras, they are extremely important, and I believe they strongly affect the working of the chakra system as a whole. They are closely involved with our connection to the earth, for if they are blocked, the head (along with the rest of the upper part of the body) becomes disconnected from the legs and the feet. Then the energy in the upper part of the body cannot move down and the energy in the lower part cannot move up. When these pelvic chakras are blocked, the whole pelvis becomes blocked, which will block the first two chakras as well. The reverse is also true: blockages in the first two chakras will block the pelvic chakras. Therefore, it is no surprise that many of the same emotions that block and get stored in the first two chakras will also block and get stored in the pelvic chakras. This includes fear, sexual programming, and emotions having to do with intimacy. Even the shoes we wear, because of their effect on our pelvises, tend to cause blockages in these chakras. In Jin Shin Jyutsu, the points that correspond to these areas of the body are called "joy and laughter" points. When our pelvises are blocked, true joy and laughter become impossible. Orange is a good color for opening these chakras.

One of the most important things to remember about the chakras is that although they each have their individual functions, they work together much as the stomach and the intestines work together, and a block in any chakra will affect the whole system. (Read Appendix C, at the end of the book, for more information on the chakras.)

When we do the aura balancing, we will also make use of some of the lesser chakras. Every joint can be considered a minor chakra, and we will use the shoulders, elbows, and knees, as well as the chakras in the hands and feet, for the balancing.

COLORS IN THE CHAKRAS

Historically, there have been many conflicting opinions about which colors are predominant in each particular chakra. My own interpretation is that the colors in the chakras can vary. A chakra usually has a mixture of colors in it, and at different moments different colors may predominate. Since I am not usually interested in seeing the colors in other people's chakras (I tend to look for *information*—pictures, blockages, and so on), I cannot say how much or how often the chakras typically change colors. But during meditation I am aware of the colors that predominate in my own chakras; and since my experience does seem to fit the current consensus, I listed them in the chakra descriptions. *Use that list as a general reference, not a hard-and-fast rule.* For instance, although I would hesitate to channel red into one of the higher chakras (in general, it represents a lower vibration), if my intuition told me strongly to do this, I would. At the same time, although green isn't often found in the higher chakras, it is a neutral enough color to use in any kind of healing, so you can do a whole in-depth balancing with the green earth-energy.

In my color scheme all of the higher chakras can have white as a predominating color; they are all working with the higher Self.

THE EMOTIONS AND THE ORGANS

In the West we are just beginning to discover the connections between various emotions and the organs of the body. Doctors have developed an "emotional profile" of people who are susceptible to heart attacks and of those most likely to acquire cancer. But although it is common knowledge that animals urinate when afraid, the medical establishment has not yet documented that people who go through life in constant fear, holding a lot of unconscious anxiety in their bodies, are susceptible to kidney-based diseases like arthritis. In the East, awareness of organ-emotion relationships has long been a part of medical practice. The table describes these relationships.

Kidneys and bladder: affected by fear.

Liver and gallbladder: affected by anger and emotional frustration. The liver in particular is affected by almost any kind of deep emotional pain or frustration, while the gallbladder is particularly affected by bitterness. They both control and are affected by the eyes.

Lungs and large intestines: affected by grief. (Cancer is associated with unreleased grief and self-pity, even if the cancer isn't in the lungs or large intestine.)

Spleen and stomach: affected by worry, defensiveness, depression, and hatred.

Heart and small intestine: affected by insecurity and emotional pretense (a form of self-alienation). Deep emotional pain, when repressed, will therefore show up in these areas. People who are always on the go will also be affected in these areas because an inability to relax indicates that something is repressed—a form of pretense.

*   *   *

It is important to understand that the relationship between the organs and the emotions is reciprocal: once an emotion has started to affect an organ, the tension in the organ makes the person more susceptible to that emotion. Conversely, as the organs become relaxed and healed, the tendency to experience those emotions is reduced. Transformation can occur either through emotional awareness and letting go or through healing the associated organ.

Although the table does not apply to *all* situations—breathing concentrated chlorine fumes will damage the lungs whether there is any grief present or not—for the healer, understanding the relationship between the emotions and the body is very useful because it helps explain the root causes of many common problems. Also, if a healer perceives that a person is strongly affected by certain emotions, knowing the associated organs will direct the healer to check those organs for emotional tensions held there, and to concentrate more healing energy in the affected areas.

More and more people are becoming aware that the food we eat may not be as critical to our state of health as the thoughts we feed our minds.

PICTURES

Wherever there is tension or blockage in the body (tension and blockage are synonymous here), stored with that tension are memories of what caused it. Ten years later, if the tension hasn't been released, the memory will still be locked up in it. Therefore, occasionally when you do healing work for someone they will spontaneously remember events from the past. It is also possible, since you will be in a sensitized state of awareness, that you yourself will see this memory as the tension relaxes and lets go. Do not be disturbed by these "pictures."

They are just a sign that something is being released and that healing is taking place. As you keep channelling, the release will complete itself. Later, if it seems appropriate, you can share these pictures with the person you were channelling for. In some circumstances, you might want to share them while they are happening (but don't stop channelling while you are doing so). I think of these pictures as weather. I am not bothered by the weather; I just keep channelling.

Sometimes you won't see what the picture is, but you will sense a particular emotion moving through the receiver. This is just more weather. As you keep channelling, the emotion will be completely released. Occasionally your awareness of the emotion being released will trigger a similar suppressed emotion in yourself (even if you are not consciously aware of what the receiver is releasing). If this happens, you will not just sense the emotion releasing from the receiver but will start to feel the emotion in your own body. You may think then that you are being enveloped by what the receiver is releasing; but that is not the case. If you feel something in your own body, what you are feeling is your own Stuff. The exception, of course, is if you are simply "patterning" the receiver's release, in which case you are not lost in the emotion but are using your body to be aware of what is happening. (See Chapter 7, "The Illusion of Picking Up Other People's 'Stuff'.")

If you start to feel emotional because of your Stuff coming up, stay relaxed and detached, and keep channelling. Remember, it's just more weather. If you don't resist the weather, it will simply pass through. This is cultivating "conscious acceptance and nonreaction." But if you feel yourself getting stuck, you can always step back and clear yourself. (If you can, first wait until the receiver has finished releasing.)

You may wonder what the effect will be on the other person if you are channelling while experiencing your Stuff. At worst, this will trigger the release of some similar Stuff in the other person—which is perfect, since releasing Stuff is exactly what the receiver is there for.

EXERCISE 5: LISTENING TO A PERSON'S BODY

This is a simple exercise. Whether or not you "hear" anything, feel anything, or see any pictures, the act of listening is a good habit to get into before starting an in-depth balancing. The more blocked or traumatized an area is, the easier it is to sense that something is wrong, because the area will have a charge of concentrated energy. In addition, it will feel more resistant to your channelled energy moving through. In the beginning, you may sense only the most severe blocks, and you may encounter severe blocks only occasionally. But during those sessions you will spend more time and direct more energy where it is really needed. Eventually you will become more sensitive and able to pick up more subtle blocks.

To begin, choose which person will "listen" first. The other person will lie down on his back, on either a couch, the edge of a bed, or a table (with a pad or folded blanket for comfort). The listener can sit or stand, whichever is most comfortable.

The listener uses her hand to listen. Channel a little energy into your hand, and as you move your hand over your partner's body, sense through the energy in your hand what is happening. This is somewhat like "looking down the energy," except that you will be using a more general awareness than just looking. I call this "sensing through the energy." Use whichever hand you prefer (you can experiment). Hold it an inch or two above the body, and slowly move it over the body, being sure to cover all the organs and chakras, including the joint chakras. You can vary the speed of your movement.

You may sense variations in the body as you move your hand. Some places may feel warmer or colder, or there may be a lack of aliveness, which indicates that some kind of tension (mental, emotional, or physical) is preventing energy circulation. The block may be recent or very old. In general, the colder or less alive the area is, the older the tension. You may sense emotions in certain areas. You may also see pictures. And if you feel and see nothing, do not be discouraged. Don't try to force it. Just be open to whatever you experience.

When you are finished, try another way to listen: through the receiver's wrist pulses. Hold the inside of both wrists with your fingertips (with three or four fingers on each wrist), so you can feel both blood pulses. Imagine that the pulses are a door through which you can be aware of the energy in the receiver's whole body. You may be able to sense anger or fear or some other emotion in the person. You may feel it only through one wrist, which indicates that it is being held in that side of the body. The side that is beating harder is the side that is more physically blocked and in general needs more help. But the other side may still be holding emotional charges that need to be released, too.* Again: if you do not become aware of anything through your listening, do not be discouraged. As you practice listening, your awareness will become more sensitized.

Wait until you are completely finished listening before you share your experiences with your partner. Then switch places and let your partner listen to you.

When this listening exercise is done at the beginning of an in-depth aura balancing, you have to decide if it's appro-

---

*In general, the left side of the body represents "the generations" and the right side the "present generation." Left-sided tension is the stress built up around inherited weaknesses, including blocks and emotional patterns picked up in the womb. Metaphysically, the left side is the karmic situation we are born with. Right-sided tension is new stress created in the current generation—what we have created out of our karmic situation—which includes stressful behavior patterns we learned by imitating our parents. Often, though, physical symptoms on one side of the body are caused by stress held on the other side.

priate to say anything to the other person about what you "hear." Usually it's best to save all feedback until the end, to avoid a discussion which will interfere with the balancing. If the person asks what you are doing while you are "listening" (by now he should have his eyes closed), you can explain that you are getting a feeling for his energy.

EXERCISE 6: RESISTANCE

This is the last exercise before starting the in-depth balancing. The purpose of the exercise is to learn how to recognize when someone is putting up a block to receiving healing energy. This rarely happens, and you may never encounter it, but it is important to be able to recognize it should it occur, because no healing can take place as long as this kind of block exists. Sometimes, since the block is unconscious, simply recognizing it and asking the receiver to give you verbal permission to come into her aura will be sufficient to let the block down. Tell the receiver to say out loud, "I give you permission to come into my aura and perform healing work." Sometimes, though, there is nothing that can be done. The receiver is not "wrong" or "bad" for putting up a block; it is an instinctive means of self-protection and may be what the person needs at this time for her own survival and security. (Once I encountered this in a woman who was protecting a recent trauma she wasn't ready to deal with yet.) Sometimes it might help to talk, *nonjudgmentally*, about the receiver's need for protection. You can show her, compassionately, that you understand her desire for protection and ask her if she truly feels that she needs protection in this particular situation. Again, sometimes there is nothing that can be done. Simply respect the person's desires and tell her that you are not able to continue with the healing.

In this exercise, one of you will channel healing energy and the other one will block it. The person who is blocking will lie down (on his back) on a couch, the edge of a bed, or a padded table, and the channeller will sit on the edge of a chair or stand. The channeller then chooses the healing energy she prefers and channels it into the other person's heart chakra, while the receiver does whatever he can inside himself to block the energy and resist receiving it. The channeller should ask the resister if he is ready before placing her hands over (not physically touching) his heart chakra. Five minutes is sufficient, and then the channeller will become the resister. Do not discuss your experiences yet.

Next, repeat the exercise, except this time use a different means to block the energy: the resister simply imagines himself lying in a cocoon of protective white light that is capable of keeping out all outside energies. Remember: energy follows thought; so just believe that you are protected by this cocoon and allow yourself to feel relaxed and safe within it.

After both of you have attempted to channel through the cocoon, share your experiences. Compare how you felt utilizing the different methods of blocking energy and compare your attempts to channel through them.

11

IN-DEPTH
AURA
BALANCING

For the first few in-depth aura balancings that you do, I recommend working with the second method of channelling, using the green (or if you prefer, the white) earth-energy. There are several reasons for this. First of all, because you are sourcing through your feet, you remain *in* your feet, connected to the ground. At first, because of all the shifts in energy that occur during an aura balancing, you may get a little lost, "spacy," or caught up in your head. A solid connection with your feet gives you a rock to stand on, something solid to focus your attention on. With the other two methods, the focus is more mental. Another reason for using the second method is that it makes it easier to monitor what is happening in the receiver's body. I'll explain more about that shortly. Finally, although most of the balancing will be done with this method, at the very end there is a step where the third method is used, bringing in a deeper level of awareness and energy. The earth-energy is used to clear the receiver's aura and chakras, and then later the heart-channelling moves the healing to a deeper level. Therefore, if you use the second method, you will be working with an energy that is easy to channel for a long time, and at the end of the balancing the receiver will still resonate with the finer quality of energy represented by the heart-channelling. After you have done a few balancings like this, feel free to experiment using the other channelling methods. When you feel comfortable with all three, you can then choose whichever feels more appropriate for the needs of the person you are working with. Also, feel free to keep your eyes closed while you are channelling, just opening them to check where your hand is or to move it.

THE PRINCIPLE OF IN-DEPTH AURA BALANCING

The basic principle of in-depth aura balancing is to clear the receiver's aura and chakras, get the body's energy system balanced and circulating in a correct pattern, and then deepen the quality of healing energy flowing through the receiver. A complete aura balancing can take anywhere from forty-five minutes to an hour and a half, depending upon how deeply you clear the person (deeper takes more time) and how blocked he is to begin with. If a person is fairly clear, a good balancing may take less than an hour.

When you clear the person's aura, you will start above the receiver's head at the eighth chakra and will move the energy down through the body, clearing each chakra with it, and then moving it out the hands and feet. (This will be explained in detail.) To clear the chakras below the crown chakra, a simple way of moving healing energy is used: putting healing energy into the crown with your right hand (sometimes other chakras will be used instead), while holding your left hand above the particular chakra you want to clear and feeling the energy come out there. (The crown chakra connects to all the other chakras.)

As the healing energy moves through and out of the chakra, it clears the chakra. And when the energy reaches the point where it is flowing clearly between your two hands, it indicates that the chakra is clear and that the connection between that chakra and the crown chakra, where the soul energy first enters the body, is also clear. It is very easy to work like this. All you are doing is feeling the healing energy in your hands, with your hands spread apart and with the chakra that needs to be cleared between them. After the chakra has been cleared like this, you hold both hands over the chakra for a minute, and it charges very easily. (As you charge it, it may seem to absorb energy like a sponge, and then when it is fully charged, you may feel your healing energy "bounce back" from it.)

When you are using the second method of channelling (sourcing from the earth) to clear chakras in this way, it is very easy to monitor what is happening. Because it will take a while for the energy from your right hand to clear the path to your left, when you first hold your left hand over a chakra you will feel a drop in the energy of that hand. You will probably (not necessarily) even feel that drop in the whole left side of your body. As the energy picks up, the energy in the left hand picks up too, and when both hands and both sides of your body feel equalized, you know that the chakra is clear. This also happens with the other two methods of channelling, but the drop and pick-up in energy are not so clearly defined. With the other two methods, the change is usually just in the hand, making the shift much harder to perceive. This factor alone would make the second method of channelling the preferred choice for the first few aura balancings.

There may be times during the balancing when you will feel yourself getting off center, or losing the sense of channelling or energy flow. Always take the time to stop, shake your hands, and clear yourself.

When you finish the aura balancing and have separated

your two auras, it will be necessary to take a few minutes to completely clear your own aura, whether you've done this during the balancing or not. This will mean clearing all your chakras. (I will explain later in detail how to do this.) The purpose of the clearing is to release any of your own Stuff that may have been triggered, consciously or unconsciously, from any of your chakras during the balancing.* In general, as stated in Chapter 7, "The Illusion of Picking Up Other People's 'Stuff,' " and in "Pictures" (p. 75), staying detached and treating all released Stuff, including your own, as weather passing through you minimizes any Stuff you will need to clear in yourself at the end of the balancing.

A side benefit of clearing your own aura at the end of the balancing is that when you are finished, you will feel as if you have just received an aura balancing too.

Doing an aura balancing is actually much simpler than explaining it, so don't worry about your first attempt. You'll do fine. If you forget something or leave something out, the receiver will still experience a very deep healing. So there's nothing to worry about. That will only create trying to's, and you know there's no room for trying to's here. Just take a deep breath . . . and relax . . .

TWELVE STEPS FOR AN IN-DEPTH AURA BALANCING

For the in-depth aura balancing, the receiver should be lying down, ideally on a massage table with her left side near the edge of the table. The edge of a bed or a padded dining

---

*If you find yourself getting stuck while you are working on a particular area of the receiver, pay close attention when you clear that area in yourself—there is a good chance that your own Stuff came up from that area too.

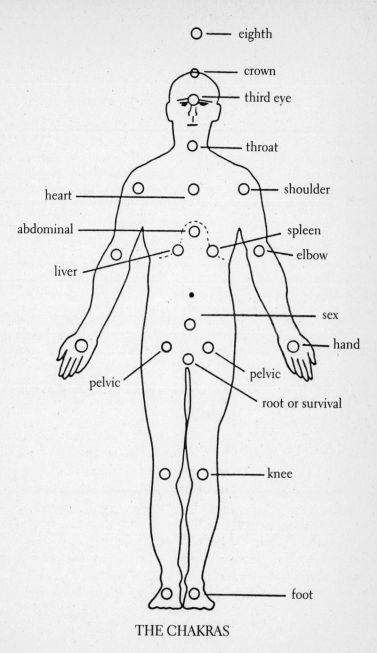

THE CHAKRAS

table is also fine. A couch can be used if there is no alternative, but the arms of the couch may get in the way. Make sure there is enough space for the channeller to sit or stand behind the receiver so the channeller's hands can be placed at the receiver's eighth chakra—eighteen inches to two feet straight back from the center-top of her head. The channeller can work standing or sitting down, whichever is most comfortable.

On the previous page is a diagram of all the chakras we will use, as well as a list of the twelve steps of the aura balancing, which you can refer to while doing the balancing.

Although I call this healing art "aura balancing," (sometimes called "chakra balancing"), it does not just involve the etheric aura and chakras. They are the primary vehicle for the balancing, but the healing strongly affects the physical body and is ultimately directed at the person—the spiritual being—inside of it. There are many ways to do an in-depth aura balancing. The method I present here is simple, effective, and creates a very deep balancing and healing.

Before You Begin: Ask the receiver if she is having any specific problems with her body. Talk to her for a few minutes and try to get a sense—without asking directly—of the kinds of emotions that dominate her life.

Step 1: Mind-Set. Once the receiver is lying down (on her back), tell her to close her eyes and relax. Explain that she may (or may not) feel unusual sensations during the balancing. Let her know that if she has the urge to take any deep breaths, or if any feelings come up, she should just allow whatever she is experiencing to happen, that it is part of the process of releasing stress from the body. If you like, gently pull on her legs and neck for a few moments, stretching them out and making them more comfortable. Then close your eyes, relax and center yourself through receiving your breath, and establish the healing mind-set.

Step 2: Listening to the Body. Hold your hand a few inches

AURA BALANCING STEPS

1. *Mind-set*
2. *Listening to the body*
3. *Connecting to the aura through the eighth chakra*
4. *Washing healing energy through the body*
5. *Clearing and charging the chakras**
6. *Specific needs (optional)*
7. *Left-right balancing*
8. *Circulating the energy*
9. *Reconnecting to the eighth chakra*
10. *Heart-channelling*
11. *Separating the auras*
12. *Clearing your own aura*

*In this order: 6th, 5th, 4th, 3rd, spleen, liver, 2nd, 1st; both pelvic; left knee & foot, right knee & foot; left shoulder, elbow & hand; right shoulder, elbow & hand.

above the receiver's body and listen for any blocks, traumas, or areas that lack aliveness. If you became aware in Step 1 of any dominant emotions, listen to the organs and chakras that correspond to them. Then listen to the body through the pulses.

Step 3: Connecting to the Aura Through the Eighth Chakra. Stand (or sit) behind the receiver's head so that when you hold your hands in front of you to feel the energy in them, you will be cupping her eighth chakra (eighteen inches to two feet straight back from the top-center of her head). Once you have taken up your position, establish the channelling, and then hold your hands in front of you and charge the air space where her eighth chakra would be (see step 3, below). When the energy feels strong, imagine the healing energy in your hands and in the eighth chakra going down to the top of the receiver's head and connecting to the rest of her body. Continue to charge the eighth chakra while you visualize and try

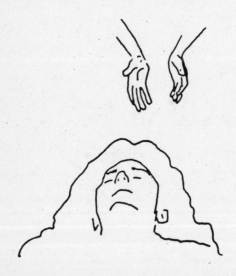

STEP 3: Charging the eighth chakra

to feel this connection. If you can't sense the connection, just visualize it, and then go on to the next step.

Step 4: Washing Healing Energy Through the Body. Move closer to the top of the receiver's head so you are holding your hands a few inches straight back from the crown chakra. (If you are using a chair you will have to move it periodically.) Your palms should partially face each other and partially face the top of the receiver's head. Channel healing energy into the crown chakra and visualize the energy going through her head, filling her whole body, and going out her hands and feet. Look down the energy and actually see the hands and feet open up as the energy goes through. (If the pelvis seems especially blocked, channel energy directly into the pelvic chakras before proceeding to Step 5.)

Step 5: Clearing and Charging the Chakras.

a. Hold your right hand an inch or two from the center-top of the receiver's head (palm facing towards her feet) while

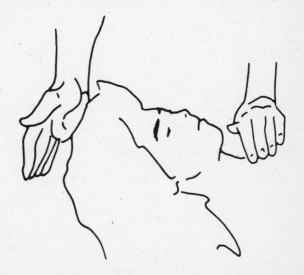

STEP 5: Clearing the throat chakra

you hold your left hand a few inches above her sixth chakra (the third eye). Wait until you feel a clear flow of energy from your right to left hand (review page 83 for what to expect here), and then hold both hands over the third eye and channel for a minute directly into it (not touching it physically). Repeat this procedure with the throat chakra, heart chakra, abdominal chakra, spleen chakra, liver, sex chakra, and root or survival chakra, in that order. (see illustration on page 85).

There will be a tendency for the right hand to move away from the center-top of the head. Be aware of this, for it is the center-top of the head that connects directly to all the other chakras. If your left hand has difficulty reaching the lower chakras that are cleared in this step, put your right hand over the heart chakra.

b. (This step is necessary, even if you worked on the pelvis in Step 4.) Hold your right hand an inch or two from the crown chakra again, and hold your left hand over the left pelvic chakra. (If this is too far for you to stretch, hold your right hand over the heart chakra.) When the energy flow is clear, individually charge the left pelvic chakra with both hands, and then follow the same procedure for the right pelvic chakra. It is very important to make sure these chakras are clear, or else the energy will have difficulty getting to the legs, and the upper and lower parts of the body will not integrate.

c. Hold your right hand above the left pelvic chakra and your left hand above the left knee chakra. When the flow is clear, charge the knee chakra with both hands. Then clear the left foot chakra (with your right hand above the pelvic chakra and your left hand above the foot.) Make sure you clear this chakra well, for this is the person's connection to the ground, and some of the negative charges that you released in other parts of the body will leave through the feet. To facilitate this release, when the foot chakra seems clear, visualize the energy going out through the bottom of the foot, and when you go to charge the chakra with both hands, visualize the healing energy going right through the sole of the foot. Then put your left hand about twelve inches out from the sole to make sure you can feel the energy coming through. (If you don't clear the foot sufficiently at first, you may react to the negative charges coming out towards your hand. The charges in themselves can't hurt you, but your reaction could get you stuck. If this happens, you can always step back and clear yourself.) When you have finished, do the right leg.

d. Hold your right hand over the receiver's heart chakra and your left over her left shoulder chakra. When you feel a clear connection between your hands, charge the chakra with both hands. Then clear and charge her left elbow chakra, and then her left hand chakra, holding your right hand above her heart chakra for the clearing phase. (If time is limited, skip the charging of these chakras.) When you have finished with her left arm, do her right shoulder and arm. (If the receiver is lying on a massage table, when channelling her right arm and leg, you can work from the other side of the table if you prefer, switching your hands.)

Step 6: Specific Needs (Optional). This step is done only if the receiver needs healing in an area that hasn't been covered. Simply channel healing energy into that area. Use whatever method of channelling you think will work best. This step is the same as "Exercise 3: Sore Spots" (see page 53). You may touch the area while channelling to transfer more energy. If the problem area is in the receiver's back, you may want to ask her to turn over, and then have her return to her original position when you have finished channelling. (For some problems the back can be reached by channelling from the front.)

Step 7: Left-Right Balancing. Now it is important to balance the left and right sides of the body in relation to each other. Hold one hand over the left pelvic chakra and one hand over the right pelvic chakra. Wait until there is a feeling of equalization. Do the same thing with the liver and spleen, and then with the two shoulder chakras. (For the shoulders, you may find it more comfortable to stand behind the receiver's head.) In this step you are not channelling into one hand and receiving with the other. You are simply allowing energy to pass through your hands and yourself in whatever direction it wants to go so the left and right sides becomes balanced.

Step 8: *Circulating the Energy.* Now energy is moving smoothly through the receiver's entire body. It is coming in the head from the eighth chakra and pouring out the hands and feet. All the chakras are clear and the two sides of the body are balanced. This is the time to circulate the energy in the specific pattern that the body needs. Stand (or sit) alongside the receiver's head, and hold your right hand behind the crown chakra as before. As you hold your hand there, look at the left foot and be aware of the energy going out the bottom of the foot. Then imagine that your hand is a kind of magnet. Visualize or feel it pull closed the bottom of the foot so the energy can't escape, and see or feel the energy being pulled by your hand up along the back of the leg, up the left side of the back and the left back of the head. When it reaches the top of the head, imagine it going back down the left front of the body, all the way to the foot, so that a large circle of energy is created going up the back and down the front of the body. Since energy follows thought, as you visualize or feel this circle of energy flowing, it will flow. It may help your visualization if you place your left hand over the left pelvic chakra and imagine that this hand is a magnet, too, pulling the energy down from your right hand and the head. Make sure you imagine the energy going *past* your left hand, though, all the way to the foot. When you have this circle of energy moving, create one on the right side, too. In Jin Shin Jyutsu, these energy flows are called Supervisory Flows; they harmonize the energy on each side of the body.

When both of the Supervisory Flows are moving, imagine a flow of energy that goes up the back and down the front of the body, this time in the center of the body, going up the spine from the coccyx and down the front, past the pubic bone to the coccyx, making a complete circle. Feel your magnetic right hand pull the energy up the spine, and if it helps, place your left hand near the pubic bone and feel this hand pull the energy down from the right hand and the head. For many people, the one hand in back of the head is sufficient to create the visualization. Make sure that the energy makes a complete circle. In Jin Shin Jyutsu, this circle of energy is called the Main Central Energy Flow. It helps the left-right balance and regulates and feeds the entire energy system of the body. Acupuncture has corresponding meridians for this extremely important energy flow. It is no accident that all the major chakras of the body, except for the spleen, lie in its path.

Step 9: Reconnecting to the Eighth Chakra. Now go back to the position in which you started the balancing—standing or sitting behind the eighth chakra. Charge the eighth chakra again, and feel its connection to the entire body. For most people, this and the following step are the most powerful moments of the balancing. This step brings the whole balancing into harmony with the soul energy, which comes into the aura through the eighth chakra.

Step 10: Heart-Channelling. The receiver is fully balanced now, and her aura is expanded and open. This is the time to take the whole balancing to a deeper level with the heart-channelling and then compact the aura a bit.

a. Establish the third method of channelling, the heart-channelling. Then channel directly into the heart chakra (without touching the receiver physically), visualizing the energy spreading out through the entire body. Feel the deepest level of unconditional love you can experience, and share that with the receiver, pouring it into her heart. Watch it fill her entire body.

b. Now imagine that the expanded aura is like a cloud. Gently gather it in with your hands, wrapping it around the receiver, compacting it a little (so she will feel more solid and grounded when she gets up), and make a cocoon out of it. Do his very gently because she is very sensitive and vulnerable now.

Step 11: Separating the Auras. Step back from the receiver now, slowly and gently separating your auras as you do so. Do not make any sudden or drastic movements.

Step 12: Clearing Your Own Aura. It is best to do this in another room, leaving the receiver to rest alone for a while.

a. Shake your hands vigorously.

b. Consciously project the thought, "All negative energy will now leave my aura." (You are the ruler of your own space.) As you think this, feel yourself let go of any negative energy that may have been triggered during the balancing. Just feel it move out of your aura to be absorbed by the air.

c. Go into the first method of channelling, the sun-energy. Open the bottoms of your feet, and let the sun-energy wash through your entire body, washing any negative energy out of it, letting it all stream out of your hands and feet. Especially make sure that your arms and hands become clear.

d. Direct the sun-energy to the chakras and joints in your body that correspond to the ones you worked on in the receiver's balancing. Feel the energy come in through the top of your head, flow into your body, and flow out through each chakra, clearing it. Use the same order as in the balancing (using only the sun-energy, not the heart chakra) to clear the arms.

e. Feel the energy equalize between your left and right hips, your spleen and liver, and your shoulders.

f. Feel the bottoms of your feet closing, and visualize the three up-the-back-down-the-front harmonizing flows circulating the energy in the correct pattern in your body.

g. Feel your balanced aura connect as a whole to your eighth chakra.

h. Feel the heart-channelling enter your heart.

i. Feel your aura become more compact.

You are now finished. Let the receiver rest for a while and integrate the healing that has taken place. It would also be a good time for you to sit quietly for a few minutes, mentally reviewing the balancing and experiencing your own body in a balanced state. Then go and wash your hands and arms (from the elbows down), letting cold water run over them for a minute. This helps to clear any remaining negative charges that are on your arms or hands, and it is also refreshing.

With your next aura balancing, try to shift colors while channelling, so you utilize on each chakra one of its corresponding colors (e.g. red for the first chakra—see p.67-73). Use white for the eighth chakra, and white, green, blue, or red (but not with inflammation) for the joints. This is the preferred way to do aura balancing with the second method of channelling.

Then do an aura balancing utilizing the first method of channelling, and then using the third.

III

THE

FOURTH

WAY

12

HEALING THROUGH ONENESS

(OPTIONAL)

The fourth way of healing works very differently than the first three methods. This is not a method of channelling healing energy; it is much more direct. With the channelling methods, you are always separate from the person for whom you are channelling. The energy is coming through you and is directed towards the other person, who is outside of you. With the fourth way, "healing through Oneness," you actually become the other person, and then *as the other person*, you heal yourself.

Healing through Oneness can be extremely powerful. There will be times when no amount of channelling will release whatever block is being held by the other person. At those times, healing through Oneness often enables a release.

Instead of working with energy, this way of healing works with *awareness*. It utilizes the awareness of Oneness: that beyond our experience of separateness is a fundamental Oneness in which all individualized consciousness is manifested. Metaphorically, although there are many leaves on the Tree of Life, they are all part of one Tree. The consciousness of the whole Tree must, therefore, exist in each part, and each part must contain within it the consciousness of the whole Tree. *

To utilize healing through Oneness, you simply shift your awareness from being a leaf to being the Tree. As the Tree, the person who needs healing is simply a part of you. Since you are all your parts, you focus your awareness on being this part of yourself. In other words, you find within your (greater) Self the place where you are the person who needs healing. As you become that person, you will be able to feel what is stuck. You will have a much greater sense of what is stuck than the person does, because you will have the benefit of both being the person and having an outside viewpoint. The next step requires some creativity. Once you know what is stuck (within yourself-as-the-other-person), you must perceive (or invent!) a way of releasing it. Ask yourself what you-as-the-other-person need to do internally to release the block, and then do it. Don't be afraid to experiment. If you try something and it doesn't work, try something else. Here are a few examples to start you off:

1. If what is stuck is an emotional charge, as the other person you can:

---

*This is what Jesus meant when he said, "I am within the Father and the Father is within me." And scientists have learned that such a paradoxical structure can exist, for they can now create holograms, three-dimensional pictures constructed with light (from holographic negatives), in which a view of the whole hologram can be constructed from any piece of the negative, no matter how small.

Another way to view this Oneness is explained in the second way of perceiving connectedness when establishing the proper mind-set: The Tree is pure Energy, and the leaves are all the forms of matter that grow out of the Energy. You are both the Energy that has created all forms as well as the particular form (or leaf) that you, as Energy, have become.

    a. allow yourself to simply release it.

    b. allow enough love (or aliveness) into that part of yourself to release it.

    c. allow yourself to experience how you would feel without that charge (which will release it).

2. If what is stuck seems more physical, as the other person you can:

    a. allow yourself to feel the emotional charge that is responsible for the physical situation and then do number 1.

    b. allow yourself to experience how your body would feel if it were healthy in this area.

    c. imagine what changes in circulation, tissue quality, and so on have to occur to effect a transformation, and then allow yourself to experience these changes.

The main thing is to be creative. Follow your intuition. You also have the option, once you have become aware of what is stuck (through being the other person), to return to one of the channelling methods, since now you will be able to channel more specifically towards the exact problem.

You may find healing through Oneness easier to learn if you practice it first within your Self. Healing through Oneness can be utilized while your hands are on the other person, while you are sitting near him but not touching, or while the other person is far away. Since healing through Oneness involves working through the awareness of your Self, you are operating at a level that is beyond time and space. The only advantage of being in the same room with the person is that if you don't know him well, having him present will give you a clearer sense of the person to look for within your Self.

For some people, a psychological block may come up in utilizing healing through Oneness. If the person needing healing has a tumor, for instance, the healer may fear allowing himself to become the other person. There may be a fear of "contamination," of patterning what the other person has and re-creating it within himself. If this fear comes up, you can either recognize it as a fear and choose to go past it (having faith that you are safe and knowing that all you can ever "pick up" is your own Stuff), or you can choose to be controlled by the fear and back off. (It really is a choice!) If you believe strongly enough that you might re-create the tumor within yourself, then indeed you possibly can, for you do have the power to create whatever Stuff *(your own Stuff!)* you believe in. (Reread "The Illusion of Picking Up Other People's 'Stuff', " Chapter 7.)

If these kinds of fears are very strong in you, then you should probably not use this fourth way of healing; your fear will prevent you from being open enough to fully experience the other person and be effective. It is impossible to create healing while you are intently resisting the person or the condition to be healed. As with the other healing methods, whatever negativity you feel afterwards is simply a reflection of your own resistance. And in this method, it will also probably indicate that the condition being healed was not completely released. If you need to, you can clear your aura as you did after using the channelling methods.

Healing through Oneness is the most subtle of all the ways of manifesting healing, for it doesn't use energy at all; it works entirely through expanded awareness. Consequently, while some people will be blocked by their fear, others will not be able to utilize this way of healing because of their inability to shift their awareness and let go of their normal sense of personal boundaries. This, too, may be due to fear, although often a person's sense of her normal personal self is just too strong to shift into a different kind of awareness. Yet people who can expand their awareness may find this way of healing exciting, for it gives them a taste of the experience of Oneness. But if you have difficulty, don't push yourself to make it work. As with the channelling methods, *trying to* will block the flow of whatever needs to happen. Just accept the impasse for now, and come back to it periodically in the future. At some point, the necessary awareness will "click" into place.

Healing through Oneness, more than any other healing tool, reminds us that when we are giving of ourselves to heal other people, we are really healing ourselves.

APPENDIX A

EXERCISE 7:

CHAKRA MEDITATION

This meditation is provided as another way in which you can use your awareness of energy and chakras to work on yourself. It will help you to activate and release emotional blocks and other tensions from your chakras, as well as to charge them and bring them into a higher state of resonance. It would be helpful to first reread the section on chakras in Chapter 10. This will make you more aware of the kinds of issues and tensions that are associated with each chakra, so you will be more conscious of what is happening within yourself during the meditation.

You can do this meditation sitting on the floor or in a chair. However you sit, it's important to keep your back and spine straight but not stiff; you need to relax to do any meditation properly.

This meditation utilizes a technique of breathing colors

into the major chakras. We will also use the two pelvic chakras, since the pelvis acts as a foundation for the upper chakras and (when open) automatically connects the legs to the torso, promoting wholeness as well as creating a pathway for emotional release from the upper chakras. In meditation, the use of color tends to activate emotional blocks and other tensions in the chakras, bringing them to the surface where you can become aware of them and, by breathing into them, let them go. When more than one color is traditionally found in a chakra, it is sometimes useful to try breathing into the chakra each of its colors, as different colors may resonate with and trigger different blocks.

THE MEDITATION

1. With your eyes closed, become aware of the area of your left pelvic chakra. Breathe into this area, as if your lungs were actually located there. Visualize your breath going into this area, and at the same time feel the breath filling it up. Now, instead of visualizing/feeling that you are breathing air, imagine/feel that you are breathing *orange light* into the chakra. Keep doing this until you feel the chakra clear. One sign of it clearing is the sudden feeling of a smile or a light moving through you, originating from the chakra. You may also feel a sense of openness or space. This will always indicate that at least part of the chakra has cleared. The deeper or more completely you experience the smile, light, openness, or space, the deeper the clearing. If you feel any tension, discomfort, or emotional ill-ease, this is an indication of something that is stuck. Don't avoid these feelings; rather, try to locate the source of the feeling and breathe orange light directly into it. Because of the affinity of orange for the pelvis, orange light will tend to activate whatever is stuck here, bringing it to the surface where you can breathe it clear. When you are finished with the left pelvis chakra, do the same with the right one.

2. Breathe *red light* into your first (root) chakra, until you feel it is clear.

3. Breathe *red-orange light* into your second (sex) chakra, until it clears.

4. Breathe *green light* into your abdominal chakra. (Optional: when it feels clear, breathe yellow light into the chakra, and see if this color activates any more blocks.)

5. Breathe *pink light* into the heart chakra. (Optional: try gold light, white light, or raspberry light.)

6. Breathe *blue light* into the throat chakra. (Optional: try white or silver light.)

7. Breathe *indigo light* into your third eye. (Optional: try blue, purple, or white light.)

8. Breathe *violet light* into your crown chakra. When this chakra clears, you may suddenly feel a rainbow of colors light up the chakra, which is a reflection of its connection with all the other chakras and colors. You may also feel some other kind of sudden burst of energy, since with the clearing of this chakra, all the chakras receive more energy and come into a new alignment and resonance. (Optional: try white light.)

9. Breathe *white light* into your eighth chakra. Here, too, you may feel a sudden burst of energy.

Now, as you continue to breathe, sit quietly for a few minutes (or longer), and experience yourself in this charged, resonant, and open state.

To go deeper with this meditation, when you have finished the above instructions, including the quiet meditation at the end, simply repeat the meditation, beginning again with the pelvic chakras, receiving the breath and light more deeply into each chakra than you did the first time.

APPENDIX B

AN ALTERNATIVE

THEORY OF

DISEASE

Disease is an imbalance of the body's energy system. A body is imbalanced when some of its energy pathways are blocked, causing cellular, organic, and systemic stagnation, which is sometimes food for viruses and bacteria. *Viruses and bacteria do not cause disease, they feed off it.* Although a virus in one body can, through coughing, kissing, sexual intercourse, and so on, be spread to another, if the second body is free of the imbalance and stagnation that is food for that particular kind of virus, the virus cannot take hold in it.*

*Experiments performed by injecting healthy animals with concentrations of viruses or bacteria and causing them to become sick do not prove anything about the nature of disease, for this is not how disease occurs naturally. An analogy is the story of an Easterner who went West, and when he saw vultures eating dead carcasses assumed they had killed the animals. When people who lived in the West insisted that vultures don't kill live animals,

Once this concept of disease is really understood, the standard Western medical model for treating disease begins to look somewhat incomplete. I often hear of babies being given one antibiotic after another for ear infections. The mother simply shakes her head and says, "Whenever my child stops taking them she gets sick again." Yet it never occurs to her that the child doesn't get well because the *cause* is not being dealt with. The prescribed medication kills the bacteria that are feeding off the disease, but as soon as the antibiotic is withdrawn, more bacteria stream in to feed.*

Many kinds of disease (imbalance) do not feed viruses or bacteria, but cause physical weakness or pain. Migraines, arthritis, nausea, and ulcers are all *symptoms* of this kind of disease. Here, too, if the symptoms (e.g., migraine) is perceived as the disease itself, prescription drugs will be used which will have some effect on the symptom (as well as causing side effects), *but will not cure the disease.*† A simple example of this was a woman who came to me for help with chronic migraines after her doctor decided to inject cortisone—a very powerful drug—into her neck and shoulders to force them to relax. In addition to the side effects of the cortisone (including suppression of the body's immune system), this "cure" would have been only temporary since it addressed the symptom of her disease, not the disease itself. (Eventually the effect of the cortisone wears off, requiring another shot—a stronger shot, since the real disease, left unattended, has grown worse. Often a more severe condition will develop—see footnote, page 61.)

---

he decided to prove he was right: he captured a hundred vultures and put them in a cage with a small live animal. What do you suppose happened?
*It is important to point out that if you don't have access to reliable natural ways of treating such diseases, this vicious cycle of continuous antibiotic treatment may be your only alternative.
†Since all prescription drugs have side effects, any use of them to "cure" disease causes other problems, indicating that the Western medical model's understanding of disease is fundamentally incomplete.

My healing work with her revealed that energy pathways in her pelvis were blocked, and when these were cleared her headaches disappeared completely. Typically, the energy blockage responsible for physical symptoms will be in a different part of the body then the symptoms themselves—hence the absurdity of treating symptoms as the actual disease. This false belief that the symptoms are the disease also gives rise to the illusion that drugs heal. But *only a person's natural life force can create healing*, and therefore healing can only be *facilitated* through increasing the person's vitality, awareness, energy flow, or willingness to experience love.

Ultimately, of course, the best cure for all disease is preventing it. Therefore the next logical question is, how do the energy pathways originally become blocked? They become blocked by physical, mental, and emotional stress. And what causes us to live in ways that generate these stresses are our attitudes and beliefs. For instance, if you believe you should become angry when a car cuts you off, when your boss fires you, or when you hear something you don't like on the news, then you will create stress for yourself in the form of anger, which will block your energy system. The fact that you think it is natural to become angry in such situations is simply an indication of how deeply you believe in anger. If you believe it is natural to worry about the future, your children, or your job, then you will choose to worry and block your energy system with it. Worry is always a choice, in spite of the fact that it is often a reflex reaction. Originally, you learned to worry (you learned this well)—and you can unlearn what you've learned. You can make different choices. Worry, fear, hate, anger, pretense, self-protection, and grief are the dominant attitudes we have been programmed to believe in by our culture and our parents. I call them "attitudes" because they are learned behaviors used to define our relationship to an experience *after* it has occurred. They are boxes we put our experiences in. The day (or minute or second) after a bus splashes mud on you, you put it in a box and label it "something to be angry about." Yet the moment it was happening, you were simply shocked. The anger was a choice you made after the incident happened. You added the anger to the experience; it was not a fundamental part of the experience itself. You could have chosen to add something else—you could have decided it was funny—or you even could have had the experience by itself, without any attitudes attached to it. The latter possibility is called Being Here Now. When you are Being Here Now you directly experience Life itself; when you imprison your experience in labelled boxes, you resist Life and experience only your attitudes towards it.

As you can see, the issue of disease is really a spiritual issue, since the root cause of all your diseases is YOU. Your own beliefs and attitudes block your energy system, causing your imbalances and diseases. The disease is an expression and reflection of yourself. You alone are responsible. Therefore, working on yourself emotionally and spiritually is ultimately the only way to cure yourself of the roots of disease. And working with your energy system is a way of working on yourself emotionally and spiritually, since your thought patterns are energy patterns. The programmed thoughts, beliefs, and attitudes that make you resist your experiences in life are in themselves stresses. As you release these stresses and blocks from your energy system, your way of dealing with life changes. I've seen this happen over and over again in my healing practice. As people's energy systems come more into balance, they become freer of the reflex programming that had been running their lives and begin to see the world in a clearer way. It should come as no surprise that as people become more relaxed, balanced, and free, they also become more free of disease. No prescription drug can give you this kind of health.

As to inherited disease, in the deepest sense this inheritance

includes not only the particular physical body we are born
with but also our particular parents with their attitudes and
beliefs, as well as the culture we are born into with all of its
biases. What we inherit is the whole situation we are born
into. And since this is not, for anyone, a fully enlightened or
balanced situation, we all begin with some existing imbalance
in our energy systems. In my understanding of reality, whatever
blocks we are born with are a reflection of what, on a soul-
Self level, we have decided we need to work on in this life.
We choose whatever situation is most suited to facilitate our
growth. My next book, on personal transformation, will explore this in depth. Here it is enough to state that inherited
disease is an expression of deeper levels of your Self. You are
still responsible for the imbalances (or transformation) you
create.

In this context, epidemics may be seen as group expressions—issues that the society as a whole is dealing with. (And
on the physical level, the spread of the epidemic disease will
be easy, for with issues that concern the general society, most
people will be imbalanced and stagnant in those areas.) A
disease like AIDS, therefore, will have emotional, social, and
psychic issues surrounding it that reflect modern times. Another consequence of this point of view is that as long as our
soul-Selves need to explore growth issues through disease conditions, we will be born with sufficient imbalances to perpet-
uate disease. and if we manage with drugs (or vaccines*) to

---

*Vaccines once seemed the panacea for all diseases. Unfortunately, recent
research indicates that vaccines, which artificially stimulate the immune
system, tax its resources and weaken it, leaving it more susceptible to other
diseases. *Omni* magazine (July 1987, p. 20) reports: "Recently, researchers
at Roswell Park Memorial Institute in Buffalo, New York, discovered that
repeatedly immunized animals are more susceptible to attack by the AIDS
virus. . . . [The interviewed researcher] speculates that there may be a link
between the U.S. policy of mass inoculation and the recent rise in au-
toimmune diseases." In addition, as the number of inoculations you receive

prevent certain kinds of viruses from living off our stagnant conditions, new ones will appear—just as the AIDS virus seemed to suddenly appear. (To the medical profession these will be new diseases, but from the point of view presented here they are simply new expressions of the same imbalances created by worry, fear, hate, anger, pretense, self-protection, and grief.)

Disease has a spiritual purpose: it enables us to see where we are out of balance and forces us to grow.

---

increases, the odds of having a bad reaction to one of those vaccines rises dramatically, and just one bad reaction can cripple your health. This is not to say that vaccines should never be used, but we should be alerted to their dangers and the consequences of our current public health policy of indiscrimate mass inoculation. (Homeopathic medicine, which has long recognized that vaccines weaken the body, offers remedies to help counteract their ill effects, even if the vaccines were administered many years ago.)

APPENDIX C

POST NOTES

This section was written to answer questions that have arisen in workshops and that I have received in the mail since the original publication of this book.

HEALING ENERGY CAN STIR THINGS UP

It is important to know that healing energy can stir a person up inside—emotionally, spiritually, and physically. Old suppressed feelings or even injuries may come up; a new sense of self may emerge; the body may feel strange—or even a little sick, if some deep issue begins to release but does not let go completely. And although people want to be healed, they are often afraid of experiencing old—or even new—feelings, or disturbing the status quo in their lives.

Occasionally, a very tense person will feel a little sore after a session, because when a body relaxes, the aching that had been created by and locked into the tension comes to the surface. (This is similar to what happens when someone over-exercises: he won't usually feel sore until later, when he relaxes.) For the same reason, an exhausted person who has been pushing herself may first notice her fatigue after a healing session has energized her enough to relax and to let the deep fatigue come to the surface. (Because very tense or exhausted people may falsely think that the session made them ache or feel tired, if I am aware of their condition I will warn them about these effects beforehand.)* Even a recent injury may hurt more after a healing session if the tissue had still been in shock—and therefore somewhat numb—and the healing energy released the shock. (This is similar to the pain that occurs as the numbness of frostbite dissipates.) And an effect that happens *during* healing sessions is "gurgling"—sometimes loud gurgling—in the person's intestines. Gurgling simply indicates that tension is releasing (although release can occur without this effect). Another side-effect of tension-release is heat.

DEEPENING THE EARTH AND SUN ENERGIES

When you are sourcing healing energy from the earth or the sun (the eighth chakra), one way to deepen the vibration of the healing energy is to perceive it as an unconditional love-expression of the earth or sun. For instance, if you are channelling green earth-energy, you can perceive that unique energy as a particular love-expression of the earth and as containing that love. Then, although you will still be channelling green earth-energy, your consciousness will be more

---

*In general, with exhausted people, do not channel for more than an hour You can treat them again every eight hours. Also, when you wrap a person's aura at the end of the full aura balancing, in *Step 10b* (page 94), compact the aura more so it is closer to the body.

aligned with the unconditional love at its root and the healing energy will vibrate more deeply with that quality of love.

THE NATURE OF ORGANS

In Chapter 10, I discussed organ-emotion relationships. Technically, the relationships are actually between the emotions and our *organ-energy pathways*, which are particular pathways in the body's energy system that correspond to and feed in and out of particular physical organs. Physical organs are affected by emotion only because emotion—which is an energy phenomenon—affects these organ-energy pathways.

Think of the energy system as a special kind of tree that has fruit growing directly within (as opposed to hanging from) its branches, with each branch feeding both into other branches and back into the main trunk of the tree. Imagine further that all you can see (until you develop your "psychic" vision) is the fruit. The fruit of such a tree would then correspond to our organs, for our organs are simply the physically dense expressions of particular aspects of our energy system. Problems develop in the fruit only when there are imbalances in the tree as a whole or in one of its branches—unless there is a direct physical injury to the visible fruit. (And problems in one branch can affect other branches and their fruit.) So to heal an organ, we really need to work on the tree and branches. We can do this by channelling healing energy into the chakras, or even directly into the organ, since the organ is not separate from the branch that feeds it. Although operating surgically on an organ only treats the symptom (sometimes necessary), herbs help by strengthening the system of the whole tree and improving the functions of certain branches.

CURE TIME

Unfortunately, it is difficult to know how many sessions it will take to cure a particular condition. It depends upon the depth of the condition—which includes the depth of the mental-emotional patterns that may be at the root of it—and the person's willingness (not desire) to let these old patterns go.

I have no doubt that "genetic" diseases can be cured with healing energy. Even common sense would say that if the chaotic energy of radiation can negatively change a genetic system, healing energy should be able to re-harmonize it. Our genes are like our organs—dense expressions of our energy system—but they are formed and maintained at much deeper levels of the system. This means that for a truly genetic disease to be fully cured (many diseases which are thought to be genetic are not really that deep) a considerable amount of energy is needed—possibly ten or more years of daily healing work—to penetrate to the depth of the disorder. As long as this may seem, it is much shorter than the alternative—having the "incurable" disease for life.

MORE ABOUT THE CHAKRAS

First Chakra. Although our sexuality is associated with the second chakra, the first chakra is also involved, because our sexual energy is *activated* by the energy of our physical instinct for procreation and genetic *survival*, which rises up from the first chakra. Because of this chakra's relationship to our kidney organ-energy pathways, imbalances in male-female energies will also be based here. In addition, the first chakra is the key to our human physicality, so people who are very "etheric," who have difficulty or resistance to experiencing their physicality, will usually be blocked here.

Second Chakra. In sexual relationship we almost always create etheric "energy-cords" with our partner, connecting our second chakra to theirs. These cords facilitate connectedness, bonding, and communication, yet they also contain the consciousness of our unconscious attachments. Although energy-cords can exist with any chakras, second-chakra cords are the most common. These energy-cords mostly become a problem when a relationship breaks up, for the cord will usually still exist, maintaining our sense of attachment and thus feeding any sense of loss. In my second book, *One Heart Laughing*, I give detailed instructions for releasing these cords. Yet for the most part, an awareness of the cord and an intent to let it go will release it. (Over time, they usually release by themselves.)

Third (abdominal) Chakra. The aspect of this chakra that relates to the intellect vibrates yellow, while the personal will aspect of this chakra vibrates green. Personal will encompasses all those issues concerning "my will/my way/my control." This includes those issues listed on page 69 as well as worry, hate, depression, and the stress of our personal lifestyle—our way of living and working and eating. Some of our deepest issues for this chakra arise when we believe that our personal will and power is not sufficient to get us what we think we need to survive (physically, emotionally, or spiritually), or when we are afraid to express our personal will (sometimes experienced as a fear of expressing our anger). This eventually creates a collapse of personal will, leading to depression, self-pity, and feelings of low self-worth (issues found deep in the core of this chakra and sometimes in the spleen chakra). This, in turn, will often lead to compensations for these negative feelings, the most common of which is arrogance, which is initially our attempt to be better than the self we believe we are.

There is often some confusion concerning the location of

this chakra. Although it is generally considered to be at the solar plexus, some systems locate it more specifically at the navel while other systems place it in the pit of the stomach, just below the sternum. The chakra is actually *between* these two spots. Yet each of these spots is a focal point for particular issues and energies that are within the domain of the third chakra. Therefore, it simplifies matters to think of the third chakra as having branches that extend into both of these areas. In fact, if someone is particularly stuck in one of these areas, due to whatever is going on for that person at that time, then that person's primary third chakra blockage may also be found there.

In general, the navel area is tied into third chakra issues of control and anger—which are also, specifically, liver issues—and so the navel may be considered a backup or reinforcement system for the holding of these issues in the third chakra or liver. The pit of the stomach is involved with depression, self-protection, and "poor-me" issues, issues that are related to the stomach and the spleen.

Fourth (heart) chakra. Because this chakra is the bridge from our lower self to our higher Self and is our source of Self-love, what blocks this chakra is Self-denial and Self-alienation, which is any denial/suppression/alienation of True Self. Since all "negative" emotions block our experience of Self, of Love-Consciousness, they all have an adverse effect upon this chakra. And therefore, any chronic emotional pattern will manifest a block in this chakra, even if the pattern is rooted in another chakra; in the heart chakra the pattern will be experienced as loss of Self.

The heart chakra will also reflect our sense of personal identity (which changes as our spiritual awareness expands and contracts throughout the day). If we identify our Self with our basic worldly lifestyle or our personal will, our heart chakra will resonate with the third chakra and radiate green*; if we identify with our Higher Self, with our spirituality and un- conditional love, it will resonate with the higher chakras and radiate gold or white; if we identify with our spirituality *and* with our emotionality or sexuality, the heart chakra will res- onate with the higher chakras *and* with the second one, and it will radiate pink or raspberry; if an identity with one's phys- icality—the first chakra—is added to the last identity, the heart chakra will have a little more red in it and radiate a cranberry color. By opening our heart chakra we help ourselves remem- ber who we really are, which helps release the illusionary self- identities that created blocks in our lower chakras.

Sixth (third eye) chakra. This is the vehicle of realization (of spiritual Truth), of seeing things as they are, so it is the door to Knowledge (whereas the third chakra is the vehicle for the intellect and understanding).

Spleen Chakra. In addition to some of the third chakra issues listed above, the spleen is involved in all forms of "hold- ing back." The idea of "venting one's spleen" refers to our releasing those emotions which we have held back within our spleen.

Liver. The liver is involved in all conditions of "muscle- boundedness." In addition, I have found that most people with deep body toxicity have had some kind of liver disease, even if the disease happened fifteen years or more ago. (Of course, long term smoking and overeating of meat, fried food, and junk food may eventually create this kind of toxic condition.)

Pelvic chakras: These release tensions in both the legs and back, and help the lungs by relaxing the diaphram.

---

*This is why some systems associate green with the heart chakra, although I do not consider green one of its "true" colors. I find that healing sessions tend to turn green heart chakras gold and white, returning the green to the third chakra.

RELATIONSHIPS BETWEEN THE CHAKRAS

In general, the relationships between the chakras—how they affect each other—are best understood if the chakras are thought of in terms of the issues they represent. For instance, survival fear in the first chakra can create a block in any of the other chakras. If the fear affects (or is focused on) sexuality or emotional intimacy, the second chakra will become blocked; if there is fear of anger, or if the fear generates anger for self-protection, the third chakra will become stuck; and so on. Another example is of someone dealing with an emotional trauma in his second chakra by creating anger in his third chakra, Self-denial in his fourth, and/or blocked communication in his fifth. (Blocks in the upper chakras are mostly created by blocks in lower ones, but blocks that tie into more than one chakra can be worked on from any affected chakra.)

There are many more relationships between the chakras than I can possibly describe here. As your awareness expands, you will actually see, in your healing sessions, how a block in one chakra ties into blocks in others, and by knowing what each chakra represents you will be able to intuit the person's overall issue. The key is not to memorize pages of chakra relationships but to understand the principle I have described here.

YOGA POSTURES FOR OPENING THE CHAKRAS

Many people who practice hatha yoga don't realize that it can be used to directly open the chakras. For present and future practitioners of yoga, what follows is a list of the chakras and basic yoga postures that can be used to open them:

1st Chakra: The Frog
2nd Chakra: The Cobra

3rd Chakra: The Bow or Boat
4th Chakra: The Fish or Camel
5th Chakra: Full or Half Shoulderstands, Bridge, or Plow.
6th Chakra: Spinal Twist or Yoga Mudra
7th Chakra: Headstand or Yoga Mudra

When practicing these postures, it is important to remember that simply holding them is not sufficient; one must breathe deeply and consciously within a posture to create real release within its associated chakra.

PULLING "STUFF" OUT OF CHAKRAS (AN OPTIONAL EXERCISE)

If you could not sense any blockages in the chakras in Exercise 5, skip this exercise for now; you need to be able to sense a blockage to release it using this technique.

To begin, the channeller "listens" to the receiver's chakras (as in *Exercise* 5, page 75) until he comes across a blockage. Only one needs to be found.

Then you, the channeller, should point your fingers (of one or both hands) so they are at a somewhat vertical angle, pointing into the chakra, directly at the blockage in it. Then imagine that energy is *extending* from your fingers down into the blockage, making contact with it. This extended energy should be thought of as an energy-extension of the fingers themselves. This will enable you to use the energy just as if you were using your fingers.

Next, move your "energy-fingers" in a slow circular motion (clockwise or counterclockwise), so that the blockage becomes wrapped around them. This will be like stirring a sticky fluid with a stick, making it wrap around the stick.

Then slowly begin to pull your energy-fingers out of the chakra, so that you take the sticky blockage with them. Remember that the blockage is somewhat intertwined with the chakra (which reflects the receiver's *emotional* entanglement with the block), so the chakra must release it for it to actually let go; if you move too quickly and don't give the chakra time to disentangle itself, the blockage will simply be pulled off your fingers. If the block seems pretty stuck, having the receiver breathe deeply into the chakra may help. You may actually feel, as you pull on the blockage, that the chakra is holding on to it and resisting your pull. It may feel a bit like pulling on taffy. Simply be patient. The whole procedure should not take more than five minutes if the block is willing to let go.

When you have disentangled the blockage from her aura, simply shake it off your fingers, away from the receiver. Then "listen" to the chakra to sense the change in it.

Often, you will not have pulled the *whole* blockage out; you can repeat the exercise to get the rest of it. Sometimes it is just too large or cemented in place to move at all. Sometimes you may feel that the blockage is also tied into and being held by another chakra. In that case, you can simply extend your energy-fingers through the chakra you have been working on to the other blocked one, or you can go directly to the other chakra, going back and forth if you need to.

When you are finished, exchange places and repeat the exercise, and then share your experiences with your partner.

MORE ON CHANNELLING AT A DISTANCE

If you are having difficulty using the crown chakra to channel healing energy at a distance, here are a few tricks to help you:

1. Try feeling the energy in your hands first, and then visualize the energy going *from your hands* up through your torso and out the top of your head to your partner.

2. Imagine that you are extending your *consciousness* through the top of your head to contact your partner's consciousness and body.

3. Try breathing into the center top of your head, imagining that your breath is opening and expanding this area. After a minute or two, you will feel as if the top of your head has opened, and then you can continue with the exercise.

4. Using the chakra meditation in Appendix A before the channelling may help, and it may enable you to channel a fuller, more powerful healing energy.

If you get ungrounded or "spacey" from using your crown chakra to channel at a distance, you can either enjoy the sensation or utilize the suggestions in the *Awareness Note* on page 21 to reground yourself. Sourcing green earth energy, as if you were about to channel it, is also very grounding.

THINGS TO LOOK FOR DURING THE AURA BALANCING

Energy Sensations. While you are clearing a chakra, with your left hand over it, you may feel "bumps" in the energy flow, or feel as if little energy-things are popping against the palm of your left hand. Often, you feel as if something has been physically relaxed under your hand, or you may sense emotional feelings being released, or you may sense a "smile" coming out of the chakra—clear energy always has a smile in it.

A Stuck Chakra. If you sense that a chakra won't completely clear, there are several things you can do:

1. Change the color you are channelling to a color that corresponds with that chakra (e.g. red for the first chakra).

2. Shift to the third method of channelling, sourcing from the heart, since this is a more subtle energy and will work more on the emotional holding of the blockage.

3. Continue with the aura balancing and return to the stuck chakra in *Step* 6 of the aura balancing, when you have finished with all the other chakras. (You may rework more than one chakra in *Step* 6.) Because of the connections between the chakras, clearing the other chakras helps to loosen the block in the one that was stuck.

4. Have the person consciously bring his breath to that chakra while you channel into it. (You don't need to go into a long explanation to ask the person to do this.)

5. Use the "pulling stuff out of chakras" technique, described earlier in this section, if you are able to do this. If the block still won't clear, forget about it; it may not be ready to let go.

Emotional Release. If the receiver becomes very emotional, it is best to continue to channel so that more energy is coming in to help complete the release. Yet while you are channelling, you can lovingly tell the person that what she is experiencing is safe to experience. It is also important to keep her breathing. You simply encourage her to breathe. Every emotional pattern has a corresponding breathing pattern which the person will tend to get stuck in, and this will keep the person caught in that pattern. Breathing will also help to release the fear-aspect of the emotional pattern which maintains that it is not safe to breathe/live/feel what is happening (which is a lie).

Restlessness in the Receiver. Usually, if the person receiving the healing energy seems to be getting restless, it simply means that some kind of charge is releasing or getting ready to release. But if the person begins to get restless towards the end of the treatment and stays that way, then it indicates that the person has received all the energy his or her body is able to receive and process. In such a situation, quickly do whatever is necessary to make the session complete, and then end it.

A QUICKIE TREATMENT

When you lack either the time or inclination to do a full aura balancing, clear and charge chakras 8 through 1 (starting with the eighth chakra, as in the aura balancing), including the spleen, liver and pelvic chakras, and then finish with the heart channelling (step 10 of the sure balancing).

THE UNIFIED FIELD: MORE ABOUT ONENESS

Einstein realized that all the energy in the universe is interconnected, that the entire universe is One Unified Energy Field in which each part of the Field—whether a rock or a human being—is simply an expression of the One Field at that point. No part is separate from the whole; everything is part of everything else.

One implication of this is that if any part of the Field is conscious, then the Field itself must possess consciousness, for the part could only have gotten its consciousness from the whole. And since the Field is composed of energy, *energy must possess consciousness*. So our universe—which includes all levels of existence—is really a Unified Field of *Conscious* Energy. (Of course, this is what mystics have been saying for thousands of years.)

A human being then is a unique local pattern of Conscious Energy within the larger pattern of the One Field. An ancient metaphor for this relationship is the Tree of Life. A human being is a unique leaf on the Tree of Life, but the leaf's deepest identity is the Tree itself, for although a leaf may be *perceived* as a separate structure, it is simply an expression and a part of the Tree.

MORE ABOUT DISEASE

Because energy follows thought, both conscious and un-conscious thought, for every disease, which is a particular pattern of energy, there will be a matching pattern of thoughts—in the form of self-limiting beliefs and attitudes—whether the thoughts are conscious or unconscious, whether the disease is "acquired" or "inherited." Our thoughts have the power to create, maintain, or cure our diseases. Therefore, although the receiving of healing energy will help a person to let go of self-limiting thought patterns, in many situations channelling healing energy will not be sufficient; *sometimes healing a disease will require changing the person's way of thinking.* (This method of transformation is the subject of my second book, *One Heart Laughing*.) Although you cannot heal someone of something he is not willing to let go of, you can help him to change his mind so he becomes willing to let it go.

CONCLUSION

This book has been an introduction to a form of healing traditionally known as energy channelling or laying on of hands. It is by no means all-inclusive. It is also not meant to set down iron-clad rules, but to establish guidelines. Healing is an art. It uses the laws that govern energy the way a painter uses the laws that govern color. The bottom line of healing is to trust your own instincts and intuitions.

Practicing this kind of healing work is also a form of meditation. As you practice it, your awareness and sensitivity will grow and you will begin to experience intuitions. You may even start to have "psychic" perceptions, but all a psychic does is see what is already there in too subtle a form for most people to notice. Learn to trust what is given to you.

For me, writing this book has been a little bit like giving a workshop without ever learning anyone's name. I would love to know about the experiences you have as you practice channelling healing energy. I may also be available for doing workshops in your location. Learning to channel healing energy in a workshop setting is an incredibly high experience.

My hope is that this book has given you a taste of the magic that exists within us and around us all the time. We live in a magical universe! We need only to open our eyes. I wish you hugs and laughter on all your journeys.

With Love,

Ric A. Weinman

I can be reached by writing to: Ric A. Weinman, Circle of Inner Balance, P.O. Box 42073, Tucson, AZ, 85717.

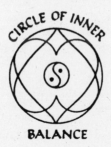

FURTHER READING

Joy's Way by W. Brugh Joy (J. P. Tarcher, 1979).

Psychic Massage by Roberta D. Miller (Harper & Row, 1975).

Creative Visualization by Shakti Gawain (Bantam, 1982).

Heal Your Body by Louise L. Hay (Hay House, 1982).

In Search of the Healing Energy by Mary Coddington (Destiny Books, 1978).

The Therapeutic Touch by Delores Kriegger, Ph.D., R.N. (Prentice-Hall, 1979).

Everybody's Guide to Homeopathic Medicines by Stephen Cummings, F.N.P., and Dana Ullman, M.P.H. (J. P. Tarcher, 1984).

Toning by Laurel Elizabeth Keys (DeVorss, 1973).

Creative Dreaming by Patricia Garfield (Ballantine, 1974).

The Nature of Personal Reality by Jane Roberts (Prentice-Hall, 1974).

Emmanuel's Book compiled by Pat Rodegast and Judith Stanton (Friend's Press, 1985).

Grist for the Mill by Ram Dass (Unity Press, 1976).

Healing into Life and Death by Stephen Levine (Anchor Press/ Doubleday, 1987).

Rebirthing: The Science of Enjoying All of Your Life by Jim Leonard and Phil Laut (Trinity Publications, 1983).

FOR THE BEST IN PAPERBACKS, LOOK FOR THE

In every corner of the world, on every subject under the sun, Penguin represents quality and variety—the very best in publishing today.

For complete information about books available from Penguin—including Pelicans, Puffins, Peregrines, and Penguin Classics—and how to order them, write to us at the appropriate address below. Please note that for copyright reasons the selection of books varies from country to country.

In the United Kingdom: For a complete list of books available from Penguin in the U.K., please write to *Dept E.P., Penguin Books Ltd, Harmondsworth, Middlesex, UB7 0DA.*

In the United States: For a complete list of books available from Penguin in the U.S., please write to *Dept BA, Penguin*, Box 120, Bergenfield, New Jersey 07621-0120.

In Canada: For a complete list of books available from Penguin in Canada, please write to *Penguin Books Canada Ltd, 10 Alcorn Avenue, Suite 300, Toronto, Ontario, Canada M4V 3B2.*

In Australia: For a complete list of books available from Penguin in Australia, please write to the *Marketing Department, Penguin Books Ltd, P.O. Box 257, Ringwood, Victoria 3134.*

In New Zealand: For a complete list of books available from Penguin in New Zealand, please write to the *Marketing Department, Penguin Books (NZ) Ltd, Private Bag, Takapuna, Auckland 9.*

In India: For a complete list of books available from Penguin, please write to *Penguin Overseas Ltd, 706 Eros Apartments, 56 Nehru Place, New Delhi, 110019.*

In Holland: For a complete list of books available from Penguin in Holland, please write to *Penguin Books Nederland B.V., Postbus 195, NL-1380AD Weesp, Netherlands.*

In Germany: For a complete list of books available from Penguin, please write to *Penguin Books Ltd, Friedrichstrasse 10-12, D-6000 Frankfurt Main 1, Federal Republic of Germany.*

In Spain: For a complete list of books available from Penguin in Spain, please write to *Longman, Penguin España, Calle San Nicolas 15, E-28013 Madrid, Spain.*

In Japan: For a complete list of books available from Penguin in Japan, please write to *Longman Penguin Japan Co Ltd, Yamaguchi Building, 2-12-9 Kanda Jimbocho, Chiyoda-Ku, Tokyo 101, Japan.*